Mount Elbrus and Mount Kosciuszko

Seven Mountain Story
Book II

Walter Glover, MTS

"How beautiful on the mountain are the feet . . ." —Isaiah 52:7

Advance Praise

"Faith, hope, and love fuel this mountain climber's passion to reach new heights."

—The Criterion, Indianapolis

"Walter's treks are inspiring to many people. It's not just the challenge of the climb at his age when most people are slowing down, but it's where his heart is while making the difficult grades."

—Bedford Times Mail

"Glover meshes with fitness as he does with prayer. He trains 120 miles per month, not simply walking or jogging but climbing any and every hill he can find while carrying a 40-pound backpack and wearing boots. One mile a day must be vertical, by the way."

—Dale Moss, The Courier-Journal
The Louisville (KY) Courier-Journal

"Glover has combined his passion for mountains with another passion, helping people, youth in particular. His expeditions to hike mountains in foreign lands are dubbed 2Trek4Kids.

—Leader-Democrat

"Wally Glover of St. Vincent's Jennings Hospital in Indiana, won the first national Eye on Wellness award from Virgin Health Miles. Wally is an active 61-year old HealthMiles member, committed to staying active and promoting activity within his community."

—Virgin Pulse
Health Miles

"Glover goes to schools and tells students the rewards of getting naturally high and healthy. He tells them they can do whatever their heartfelt passion pictures."

—The Columbus Republic

"Overcoming the mountainous battle of knocking down childhood obesity will take more than one man on a mission—it's going to take a change in society and its behaviors. However, thanks to people like Glover who point their commitment toward doing good, we know we're taking positive steps in the right direction."

—Bedford Times Mail editorial

Dedication

To Marie Meno Glover and John Glover, and their son
John Glover—my parents and brother,

To the youth and families who benefitted from 2Trek4Kids in
southern Indiana, their clinicians, and our program donors.

Contents

SECTION ONE: Mount Elbrus

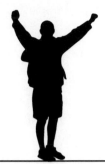

1. Mount Elbrus Highlight

*A*bout 90 minutes from the summit of Mt. Elbus, our lead guide Sergay turned to face me and announced in his clipped Russian accent, "Time for to eat."

We stood high above Russia at some 17,000 feet, near a steep outcropping that offered a break from climbing. I knew Sergey had recently claimed a new speed record up Elbrus—a huge accomplishment on one of the famed Seven Summits. This meant we were climbing with a world record holder, but he set a slow and deliberate pace for us; appropriate and doable. When I teased Sergay about how slowly he moved today, a tiny smile creased his lips.

I followed him onto the rocks and found one I could straddle, with my butt up the mountain from the rocky mass and my legs astride it. The steepness of the mountain was such that I could securely wedge my cramponed boot heels into the snow-covered icy glacier. Fairly comfortable, I felt secure with this seating arrangement. A minute later my climbing partner Lori pulled in and I helped her get safely squared away. I added slowly and carefully, "If you take off your pack, anchor it above and behind that rock." A loose pack would slide all the way back to the plateau where we'd stowed gear a thousand sharply angled feet below.

A stunning panorama lay before us. Russia's Caucasus range stretched in all directions and we were higher than all the glacier covered peaks in sight. We were also above the cloud deck, but the clouds were moving, our sunlight becoming eclipsed. I told myself this scene might have been around since Creation days, after the continental shifts, after these volcanoes bowed out to their curtain-call explosions. What a majestic timeless vista Elohim the Creator God gave us to behold. I said some of this to Lori, telling her to treasure the view in her heart. What my rookie climber friend said in response still makes me laugh out loud.

Lori quietly took in the incredible view, then turned back to me and said, "You know I'm scared of heights don't you?"

Incredulous, I almost blurted, "You're joking!" When I realized she was serious, my eyes nearly bugged out of my head.

"Yeah, at home I won't even climb on a ladder to paint the garage or clean the gutters," she added.

Realizing she meant every word, I thought better of laughing. I was torn between telling her, "Don't look down," or saying, "Maybe those clouds will move in to hide the view." Instead, I managed to mutter: "Well, enjoy lunch." An hour later I would regret wishing for clouds.

Later when I asked Lori why she decided to climb with me, she told me about the mother of a cerebral palsy patient she cared for—how the mother and her son faced their fears. This wise woman taught herself, her son, and Lori that it was okay to be scared, but we need to look what scares us in the face. The mom had a rock inscribed with *No Fear*. That thinking empowered Lori at sea level, but today at 17,000 feet she went breathless as she gazed at the world below. She said she didn't consciously hide her fear from me—she felt she could handle it by herself, and she did.

Above us loomed 1,000 vertical feet to the roof of Russia. At 18,513 feet (3.5 miles) high, Mount Elbrus towers over the surrounding terrain. High winds, cold nights, a long summit day, and unpredictable weather make Elbrus a difficult climb with a high failure rate. But things were looking good for us, with only 90 minutes of climbing to reach the summit.

While awaiting our companions James and Roxanne we munched apples, ate chocolate and cheese, and hydrated. The water tasted good—later I'd realize how good. We'd been going upward since before 4 a.m. after awakening at 3 a.m. Soon it'd be noon. I enjoyed having the pack off. Even though we jettisoned gear down below and the pack was lighter, any weight felt heavy after eight hours at this altitude.

Our companions arrived 15 minutes later, maybe longer. Nothing was said about their pace. The mountain's "aspect," how mountaineers refer to a slope's angle, was steep on the last 1,000 feet. That steepness would continue, and it slowed Jim's pace.

When everyone finished eating we prepared for the final push to the summit. Sergey pulled a tan rope coil from his backpack and stretched it out. Time for us to rope up. We each tied the rope into the harnesses we wore around our waists—attached to the climber ahead of us and behind us. The mountaineering trope is: The Brotherhood of the Rope. Sergey led, then Jim, me, Lori, and Roxie. We were now a rope team. As such our cadence, or dance steps as I called it, needed to be in alignment and timed so we all walked in synch.

Upward we went, climbing steadily while trying for roped rhythm. A wrong step would cause the ropes to go too taut or too slack. Either way, an out-of-step climber threw off one or more of his partners. I'd spent much of the last eight hours walking behind Sergey and I had his pace dialed in. Jim moved a tick slower. For a while I found myself going a wee bit fast and bumped into him. Not that I needed this brought to my attention, but Jim brought it to my attention. Sometimes with a growl. I didn't blame him. In addition to my bumps annoying him, we were all fatigued after climbing for several hours. Jim didn't need his physical and emotional equilibrium thrown off by the guy behind him. Thankfully, after a few more bumps and complaints, I adapted to his pace.

Consider our burdens: We each wore layered clothing for warmth and carried a weighted backpack. We wore 12-point crampons on our feet over big boots. For additional safety we carried ice axes to arrest a fall. Ski goggles covered our faces.

And soon we were walking into a whiteout as the cloud deck began to envelop us. Then snow began to fall. Tiny flakes like powdered sugar danced in the air; beautiful, but not exactly a walk in the park.

Bump!

"Walter—watch it!" Jim growled.

"Sorry, Jim."

When the clouds totally engulfed us and the landscape became veiled, I regretted my earlier thoughts about clouds moving in. Now, the clouds merged so perfectly with the mountain that I could hardly see where to place my feet. The snow increased as we steadily ascended. Our crampons and ice axes bit into the glacier's hard surface. Thankfully, no one slipped or fell. We each moved efficiently. There was something of a trail from the other climbers, although here on the upper mountain not another soul was in sight. Not one. Come to think of it, the last guy we'd seen hours ago was headed down—right after sunrise. He must have overnighted on the mountain.

The higher we went, the more socked in it became, with the cloud cover and falling snow increasing. But we were nearing our goal, our quest during long months of training. I felt a surge of joy when Sergey told Jim, who passed the word to me, and on down the line, "We're getting close, about 15 minutes from the summit."

The worsening conditions made it nearly impossible to see. Visibility ahead was down to 20 feet. We couldn't see the summit, and in fact the white of the mountain's surface blended into the cloudy surroundings, producing a few missteps.

Sergey paused our rope team at a compacted, level clearing. Jim closed in on Sergey, as did I, and then the women. Sergey stretched out his carbide-tipped trek pole and slowly waved it over his head. The theologian in me imagined Moses waving his staff. I started to tease Sergey, asking if he were going to part the clouds like Moses did the sea. Sergey was not amused.

Not in the mood for a Biblical reference, Sergey continued holding up his trek pole, the metallic end pointing skyward, and the handgrip near his face. He looked at me with a steely gaze and commanded, "Walter, listen."

He thrust the trek pole handle near my ear and I heard buzzing and crackling. Sergey was monitoring weather in the air, specifically electricity. The metal end of his trek pole attracted electricity and produced the static sound.

For reference, consider the legend of Ben Franklin putting a kite aloft into a colonial era thunderstorm. As the story goes, the kite string had a skeleton key tied to it and that key attracted lightening.

In the few seconds I had to process this, our climb came to a screeching and non-negotiable halt. Sergey then said: "We are in electric storm. I am sorry. I send you down with Roxanne for safety."

What the guide says on a mountain is law. We signed an agreement saying so. Like that, our Elbrus adventure came to a close. Yet, as we started down, Sergey and James continued up the mountain without us. What was up with those two, I asked myself, feeling angry and frustrated. I honestly didn't know why it was okay for them to continue upward; I never asked them.

I did know an electrical storm was serious at the top of the world. I knew I had children and grandchildren; Lori had daughters. We valued our lives, and our families expected us to come back alive. Neither of us needed to be within range of a zap-and-fry electrical storm. Sergey and James were adults, single men. They could do what they wanted.

Why was I furious? Well, who do you think is in charge of weather? I was mad at God! Why? Because we trained our butts off to be there. Because we climbed all day to be within minutes of the summit. Plus, we were raising money for a noble cause—diminishing childhood obesity. Lori and I each paid a pretty penny from our own pockets to be in Russia.

And now we were thwarted by weather, with the prize almost in reach. No summit? I was steamed at God, the ultimate weatherman.

We needed a miracle.

In the Beginning

A year earlier, after I returned from my Kilimanjaro summit, my friends plied me with questions. The most common query boiled down to "Where will you go next time and when will you do it?

And from the naysayers: "Are you done now?"

I knew a lot about the Seven Summits, having already climbed on two. My first adventure took place at Mount Everest Base Camp in Nepal at 17,600 elevation. I never intended to try for the summit—only elite mountaineering men and women dare do that. I was pleased with my accomplishment as it stood ... for a while.

And then I couldn't resist a trip to Kilimanjaro in Tanzania, Africa, and where I stood atop Uhuru Peak at 19,340 feet. Each continent on Earth contains one especially high land mass with a peak thrusting through the clouds. I had climbed on two of the seven. None of my Franciscan nun teachers in elementary or junior high school considered me a math whiz, but this was not algebra— five peaks remained.

A guy named Dick Bass first conceived of climbing the Seven Summits and in 1985, at age 56, he accomplished his goal. He scaled most of the seven with his friend Frank Wells. Bass founded Snow Bird Ski Resort in Utah and Wells was president of Walt Disney Studios. He wrote a compelling book about being the first human to stand atop each of the world's seven summits. I know. I read every page.

I mention Dick Bass because his book incubated the idea that I might replicate his feats. Realistically, I considered climbing "on" all the Seven Summits, not necessarily to the top. And by gosh— who knew? Maybe I could summit all seven mountains. And if I didn't tag the summit of each one, what a joy and blessing it would be to climb on those storied peaks and visit the home country and people of each mountain. Once I reached the top of Kilimanjaro, my next five challenges were:

- Elbrus in Russia, 18513 feet
- Kosciuszko in Australia, 7,310 feet
- Aconcagua, Argentina, 22,841 feet
- Denali / McKinley, Alaska, 20,320 feet, and
- Vinson Massif, Antarctica, 16,067 feet.

If all went well, I dreamed of returning to Everest for the summit. However, these ventures didn't come cheaply. Argentina would cost $14,000. Antarctica was estimated at $35,000. If I truly hoped to summit Everest, I could expect a whopping cost of

$65,000. I self-funded all my expedition costs; none of the money I raised for charity went to my climbs.

When the costs appeared overwhelming, I reminded myself, "Go after this quest one mountain at a time and don't get ahead of yourself." My American hero, Ed Viesturs, is one of the most successful climbers ever. He says his wife call this kind of thinking *compartmentalizing*. In the New Testament, Jesus says every day brings its own troubles or cares and we shouldn't get ahead of ourselves. *In the Old Testament the psalmist writes in Psalm 37, "Do not fret." And for emphasis, Psalms says it three different times in the first seven verses.*

Thus, I saw no reason to stress over a long range plan I couldn't possibly afford. I told myself: "I will proceed to climb one mountain at a time and must be in a position to pay as I go. I will use cash, not credit cards, and will not endanger my financial retirement." I assumed my excellent physical health was a given; how naïve this would prove to be.

As I studied the mountains on my list, Mount Elbrus in Russia floated to the top. Both the United States and Russia are in the northern Hemisphere and our common summer was an ideal climbing period for this peak. I'd summited Kilimanjaro in June 2009, so a year later was good timing for several reasons: the climbing calendar and weather were favorable; my budget had time to recover from the African expense; and I was nearing a new assignment in my work at the hospitals I served. I could do more fundraising for youth obesity at the Jennings hospital before transitioning to our two newest St. Vincent hospitals. And finally, I looked forward to training during winter and spring without suffering the heat and humidity of a southern Indiana summer.

I announced my intentions by adding a notation to my signature block on St. Vincent Jennings emails. The block carried a tag line to promote each climb destination, stating I would be raising funds for youth obesity prevention and treatment at the North Vernon hospital ministry. Everyone who read my messages would see this fund-raising and awareness-raising promo. Not many people in Indiana climb world-class mountains, so my tagline generated plenty of feedback. The fact the first climb at Kili raised $22,000 to develop the obesity program raised people's eyebrows—in a positive way. Mostly.

Lori Walton, RN BSN was one of the first people to notice the Mount Elbrus signature line. Lori was the co-founder and manager of L.I.F.E. (Lifetime Individual Fitness and Eating program) for Kids at Peyton Manning Children's Hospital in Indianapolis. This was the clinical initiative at St. Vincent to prevent and treat youth obesity in children and educate their families. In addition to herself, Lori used registered dietitians and behavioral therapists to manage and mentor patients and their families. The team had a lot to do, because one of every three Hoosier children is clinically overweight or obese.

Lori was effervescent, strong as she was cheerful. She carried before her an invisible banner about being all for kids, their health, and being innovative and bold in regard to children's fitness and nutrition. A Hoosier from Indianapolis, she attended classes at Indiana University, Bloomington and then matriculated to Indy to receive her RN, BSN. She was mentored by a St. Vincent Carmel associate who recognized her potential.

Lori moved to the emerging Peyton Manning Children's Hospital at St. Vincent as St. Vincent set roots in this discipline. In some ways Lori reminded me of my beloved Aunt Angie Meno. Both were overweight as children. Aunt Angie overcame her issue with a combination of faith and will. Lori had those attributes—plus her knowledge of science through nursing. Aunt Angie influenced me and others by imprinting the values of nutrition and exercise. Lori did the same, adding education and clinically teaching wellness to thousands of children and their parents through her clinics at Peyton Manning Children's Hospital at St. Vincent, and by bringing her program to my hospitals at Salem, North Vernon, and Bedford.

The plan was for Lori to model the St. Vincent Jennings' program after the excellent program she helped develop in Indianapolis. So Lori became our "go to" person. As we imported her program, she would teach our staff how to adapt it to our hospital and market. I sat in on the formation meeting with our clinical staff as a liaison for the Hospital Foundation, the sponsor of my climbs which raised money to fund the program. Lori generated enthusiasm with her clinical experience, program success, and confidence. We were well begun.

As Lori and I exchanged emails and phone calls about the new program, she noticed my signature. "What's this Elbrus on your email signature?' she asked the next time we talked, which was in October.

"It's a mountain in Russia, and like the signature says I'll be going there in June," I said. "The trip will help me raise more money for the Jennings youth obesity program."

After a brief pause when I could almost hear the wheels turning in her mind, Lori said, "I'd like to do that too. I haven't raised a dime for youth obesity. This would be my opportunity to do that. Plus, it sounds like a great adventure. And I have a dream to get my program at all the St. Vincent hospitals. Maybe you can help me with that."

As for the trip to Russia, I wasn't so sure I wanted company, yet I hated to say no. I stalled, saying, "We should both think about this." Then I offered a number of tactful reasons to discourage her. She persisted. Finally, we agreed to meet for dinner and talk about it.

We met in Greenwood for dinner, only the second time we were together. An inch or two shorter than me, Lori was attractive, and athletic looking. Black curly ringlets of hair framed her joyful countenance. Remembering her from Jennings, I realized she had a penchant for black clothing that matched her hair. I expected her young patients took an instant liking to her because she was friendly, engaging, and smiled a lot. When she ordered dinner I learned Lori didn't eat red meat and liked vegetables.

When we sat down, right away I asked about her physical performance resume. Lori told me about her accomplishments: Two marathons, two bicycle Rides Across Indiana (the 150+ mile ride from Terre Haute to Richmond), and many Indianapolis mini marathons.

Lori spoke with great enthusiasm, telling what she did. Though not immodest, it was apparent she liked Hoosier-style adventures. She didn't over-reach in her story telling. She did talk fast when she got excited. And I heard the word "amazing" more than once. She seemed to be pleasant company—and she could hold her end of the conversation without going into monologue.

Still, I wasn't convinced. This was all fine as far as it went, I supposed. I just didn't know. I had easy reasons to say no. She'd never been on a mountain, didn't experientially comprehend elevation, had never been on an expedition the scope of what Russia would represent, no travel outside the US, and I just didn't know her that well. (I didn't even know she was afraid of heights).

Still, I had a dream of mountains and was acting on it. And Lori was key to the development and success of youth obesity at St. Vincent, including getting it under way at Jennings and possibly at the new hospitals—Salem and Bedford. Her friendship and participation would be a valuable connection. Moreover, who was I to piss on someone else's dream?

I found a reasonable balance point. "Tell you what. I'll let you train with me for six weeks. Let's see how you do and how we get along. It will be pass-fail, and I'll make the call."

Yes, I know this sounded arrogant and controlling, as Lori would later remind me. But I didn't want to endorse something unless it had the likelihood of success. Nor did I want to sign off on something unsafe. The mountains have zero tolerance—no room for mistakes. People have died on Mt. Elbrus. Plus, selfishly I wanted the summit. I didn't want to hold someone back or be held back. In the end, my decision was about prudence. "Did Lori belong on an expedition to an 18,500 foot mountain half a world away?"

Lori had her own considerations and strategy. She told me later: "It's a free country. If you said no and I believed I was good to go, I planned to sign up anyway."

We trained every weekend for six week ends. We took long hikes with heavy backpacks at Brown County State Park in Nashville, 16 miles west of my home in Bartholomew County. We also trekked up and down hills in western Bartholomew County where Brown County's upland extends east into Bartholomew. Our treks included the hilly neighborhood and environs inside Brown county where my son and his wife Jill lived. Lori stayed right behind me every step of the way. Whenever I turned around, Lori was proving her mettle. Plus, she stayed positive and upbeat.

Lori had listened to me about climbing clothes—boots and most gear, but she bought a backpack before I had a chance to look at it, and it didn't fit well. She constantly adjusted the shoulder straps. She wanted to be warm, so she took all the necessary precautions to ensure that. She was vigilant about drinking water. Her key attributes were fitness, a positive attitude, good humor, and physical strength.

"You're the strongest woman I ever met," I told her at the end of six weeks as we ate a meal after training. I added, "Congratulations. You passed."

She accepted my congratulations with a nod and a smile. And, that's when I remember being told I was arrogant and she'd already made plans to go without me, if necessary. We both laughed. *Look out, Russia*, I thought. *Here come the Hoosiers!*

Lori took our training seriously. On her own she flew to Colorado to meet an RN friend from Indy who had migrated west. They went climbing on Pike's Peak together—one of Colorado's fifty 14teeners. I'd already given her a passing grade; now she received extra climbing credits for an A+.

We continued training, sometimes together on weekends, and individually. We went out in snow and unpleasant conditions—as far as they go in Hoosierland. Lori always held her own. A good thing, because Russia was going to deal us onerous and dangerous mountain weather the likes of which she'd never seen. Not to mention the elevation—3.5 vertical miles high.

MARCH – MAY 2010

Our training continued and intensified. Trip preparations were commenced and finalized six to eight weeks out. Flights, Russian visas, arrangements with the trek company, insurance, equipment purchases, as well as rental equipment arrangements were all in place. I learned early that navigating Russian red tape was complicated and expensive. There also was packing, unpacking, and repacking.

Thursday, June 17, 2010

We were mere days away from departure.

Early morning call: My dearest friend in the world Kit's dad was dying, and Kit called to tell me. He said he talked to his siblings and they all wanted me to preside at the funeral. I said I would do it and delay the Russia expedition.

"No, don't do that," he told me.

I knew his dad, "Blurp." And I felt so pained that I couldn't be two places at once. But Kit insisted I stay with the mountain timetable, and I was grateful to be excused. Still, guilt feelings and authentic tension gnawed at me. Being asked to preside was an honor and a gift—a gift I had to refuse. Yet, Kit was so kind about it. How wonderful to have an understanding best friend and be excused without judgement.

A day later my emotions swung the other way as the time for departure arrived. Before departing to climb mountains I always had a Farewellin event—a festive practice I learned from completing mountain expeditions in foreign lands. Before returning home from the country where you climbed, your in-country hosts gave you and all their climbing visitors a sendoff party they called Farewellin. These were joyous celebratory occasions and also reflective. You were leaving your hosts and likely saying farewell to expedition companions you wouldn't see again. With them, on difficult terrain, you had given of yourself amid the beauty and altitude on some of the highest mountains on earth. Bonds of friendship were forged, yet separation loomed ahead.

I so appreciated the celebratory experience that I imported it to Indiana as a kind of pre-departure Hoosier Hospitality—throwing a party for myself and my friends at home. What a blast we had at this Elbrus Expedition Farewellin event! So many wonderful people made the Russian send-off a great evening. People came from across the state and across my street; family, folks I didn't get to see too often, and a host of Columbus friends. What a celebration. Did I count thirty attendees? Maybe more.

The most beautiful 14 month old in the world, my granddaughter Siena Grace, arrived in a red wagon in the company of my son Dominic and his wife Kathryn. Son Andy and his wife Jill were present. We overflowed the verandah and into the backyard on a lovely late spring evening.

My favorite story from the gathering involved Jane Richardson, a friend from my high school lifeguarding days in Bedford, Indiana many years ago. Jane and I had recently re-connected at the St. Vincent Seton Cove Spirituality Center on the Indy hospital campus. On arriving Jane told me excitedly, "At lunch today I was talking to a friend of mine and I told her: 'What I'm doing tonight will surprise you. I'm going to go visit a friend in Columbus from my Bedford days who's crazy enough to climb a mountain in Russia'.

"My friend, who's also named Lori, looked at me strangely and said, 'Oh, my God, I know about that. The woman going with him is the sister of the guy I date.'"

Once again, I realized it's a small world.

St. Vincent in Indianapolis was represented in another extended way that evening with Information System's Jeff Scott's parents attending. Jeff was regularly at my hospital ministry at Jennings in his extended geographic responsibilities to provide IS coverage from Indy. Jeff's parents Myra and Roger had just moved from North Carolina to Columbus. We'd met and here they were. Indiana University college buddies Mark Fritz and wife Deb journeyed from Indy, and Dante Raggio, and Mary K from Muncie. The Columbus entourage included Haros, Eckerlys, Heldts, Scherschels, Dana our pizza chef extraordinaire, Colleen, Josh and Jessie, Steve Thomas, and apologies to those I missed who took time to say: "Be Safe, best wishes" and "Climb that mountain!" I especially enjoyed re-connecting with my friends from Bedford, and introducing them to others.

I slipped cards to Dom for his birthday and wedding anniversary as these would occur during my absence in Russia.

Our group laughed and feasted on Dana's pizza and beer in the hot, mildly humid Indiana weather. Hugs and laughter, pizza and beer—what could be better?

Lori arrived late, after an early morning of last minute packing followed by a hospital clinic day with a late afternoon of patients. Family and friends soon began to leave for the long drive home, but several couples lingered to continue laughing and talking as the glow of the pre-solstice sun softened in the west. Then it was time to clean up. Dawn and departure would come early.

I had neither angst nor fretting, but in the back of mind, amid the anticipation, lingered an awareness that ahead of us lay a world-class undertaking on a mountain that had claimed many lives by crevasse and capricious weather. I offered a prayer for our safety.

Friday, June 18, 2010

Travel Day

We arrived on time to the Indianapolis Airport, and to our gate. That morning resumed where the previous morning left off—a talk with Kit about his dad's circumstances. I spoke to Kitter of my prayers and I offered them over the telephone. He told me to climb the mountain well.

I checked my St. Vincent Blackberry for any last minute pre-flight info. Oh, my. A friend from St. Vincent Jennings was asking me to preside at the funeral of her sister-in-law in Bedford. The woman, a hospice patient who just died, was someone I twice visited at home. The patient and I connected, as I did with her husband, who was the brother of my friend at St. Vincent Jennings. I emailed my apology and appreciation for being asked.

I shook my head, feeling emotional from these two end-of-life conversations. I went a little wobbly. I needed to *center down* as the Quakers say, getting into that sacred space of inner quiet to open up pathways to God amid disquiet. And, while waiting at the airport gate, I did so.

At last, they called our flight to Kennedy Airport in New York City. The flight wasn't long by clock time, but my soul felt enriched by the quiet minutes. I was refreshed. The flight over to NYC was short and seamless, with a brief time on the ground at JFK. Soon we boarded another flight—this time for Moscow. As we went airborne, I journaled, "Can this really be happening?" Both a question and a statement of wonder.

Lori busied herself settling in and getting comfortable. We both wore our hiking boots, which were comfortable, provided support and safety for our feet lest our most important toes get stepped on, and saved packing space. Lori took the boots off. She situated her airline pillow, saw I wasn't using mine, and asked if she could; I complied. We talked excitedly about our trip, and before we knew it the stewardess served beverages and dinner. We were both tired and talked out for the moment. Lori paged through some magazines, including a couple on fitness she'd bought at the airport. She started a movie, but soon had her chair tipped back and fell asleep. I had the aisle seat and she was next to me in a five person center row.

In mountain environments I always make safety a priority. This time I felt the added responsibility for someone else—Lori. I wanted to ensure her well-being without micro-managing our trip. Of course, she said and believed she was responsible for herself. Good for her, and I admired her strength, determination, and independence. However, as the one with mountain experience, I saw myself as what I jokingly called the climbing leader. This wasn't about control. I don't have that problem and I listen to others who know more than me. Looking ahead, I wished for that listening attribute from Lori when I made calls to keep us safe.

Our jet from JFK to Moscow seemed to follow the rising sun's arc through the sky, seen from the windows of our plane. For me, sunrises have long been what I consider hallelujah moments—a time to joyously and generously praise God. I'm not much of a singer, as the teaching nuns from my childhood would tell you if they were alive. But sometimes the sunrise praise overcomes me and I even sing aloud.

The translation of the compound word *hallelujah* from the Hebrew language means *praise Yah*. We are told ancient Jews were forbidden to speak God's complete name—*Yahweh*. Simplistically speaking, ancient theologian or rabbinic teachers of that early era assigned God, or Yahweh, a nickname, as it were. Their construction of "hallelu" for "praise" was joined to the nickname for God—*Yah*, a shortened form of the name of God from the letters YHWH, by which the Jewish people referred to God without naming Him. The psalms, particularly 113 through 150, and in Exodus Chapter 15, frequently use this construction. Thus the Jewish people avoided the trespass of saying God's name. The result: Give joyous praise in the name of the creator God.

Hence the phrase *Hallelu Yah!*

This action to praise God's name, coming from the ancients writing the Old Testament, energizes me. Sunrise, sunset, special events, and ordinary occasions invite me to echo Hallelujah! Usually with feeling. Pope John Paul II now canonized a saint, referred to the Jewish people as "our older brothers in faith." They were and are a faith people who eloquently use language to glorify God.

On this section of the trip I found many opportunities for Hallelujah moments. Flying east we watched the lengthening sunrays illuminate our aircraft. Kodak moments unfolded and Lori recorded them with photographs.

Over Iceland we saw smoke and debris rising toward our wings from a volcano whose eruption had earlier threatened our travel plans. The volcano's name is Eyjafjallayokull. Really. Try saying that in one breath—or saying it at all. The eruption spewed a threatening amount of ash thousands of feet into the air. The view below appeared to our Western eyes like the volcano produced a huge mess. Tens of thousands of people in Europe were stranded for weeks, unable to fly to or from airports. Some airlines cancelled flights for as long as a month because of danger from the ash fouling airplane engines.

Worldwide there are currently 1,500 active volcanos. During our flight, ash of the volcano with the funny name had diminished and no longer threatened flights over this route. Yet we could still see it smoking.

That reminded of the psalmist writing of the Creator God, Elohim in Hebrew: "You look at the mountains and they smoke." And another: "In your presence the mountains melt like wax." Watching the active volcano below as we flew over, I made a mental mote to self: Research erupting volcanos in the Holy Land at the times of the ancients to see what volcanos the writers and people might have seen erupt, and "melt." I didn't know of any—were there? And if not, how did the ancients know to so write? Hmmm.

Our flight went on and on. Finally I slept—uncomfortably. Lori seemed to be a good airplane sleeper and did so much of the way. We were 33,000 feet above the ocean and would arrive at about 10 a.m. Moscow time.

Saturday, June 19 2010

Another Travel Day

My morning prayer for many years has been: "I will greet the new sun with confidence that this will be the best day of my life." I prayed for a few days into the future that Lori and I might see the Creator's sunrise from Mount Elbrus' peak. On a sun-filled day from the peak, I hoped to look in one direction and view the Caspian Sea, and the other direction for a view of the Black Sea.

Finally, the interminable flight neared its end and we were on approach to Moscow with sunshine flooding through the cabin windows, 9.5 hours after departing from JFK. We would land at the biggest of Moscow's four municipal airports. "I hope our pilot finds the right one," I told myself, not realizing how profound that random thought would become in our future.

Our flight was populated with an international crowd. The American element included a number of students from The Ohio State University, some of whom I visited with. An alumnus of Indiana University, I recognized OSU as a Big 10 Conference athletic foe in football and basketball. We teased about that and talked in a friendly Midwestern way. The passengers were courteous to each other and airplane friendly. If somebody coughed or sneezed it was done into the crook of the elbow. All that would change once we deplaned. Instead of the home dialect, we heard Russian spoken in an overbearing way, reminding me of military drill sergeants—except these were civilians. Signs printed in the cryptic Cyrillian language were far beyond our pronunciation and understanding. Strangers avoided making eye contact with us. Dense cigarette smoke pervaded the airport, creating localized smog for which no warning was issued. The pedestrian pace was fast and purposeful. I am no stranger to international airports, but Moscow was something else again. I wasn't sure if we were seeing civil or military armed guards here and there, but they stood out. Lori looked at me as if to say—"What's that line from Oz? 'This isn't Kansas, Dorothy!'"

Our passage through Russian customs was uneventful, other than having our health imperiled by more cigarette smoke everywhere we turned—and we stood within that smog cloud as the customs line moved slowly forward. No such thing as smoking bans in Russia. And the strong Russian tobacco smelled awful.

We had a 24 hour layover in Moscow and several things to sort through. Travel fatigue and sleep deprivation impaired my clarity of thought, and I had a little trouble focusing. We needed a plan. First we bussed from the huge main terminal to the Aeroflot Terminal where our flight to the Caucausus Mountains would originate. We exchanged United States dollars for rubles. Then we found a baggage storage business and jettisoned our backpacks and suitcases.

Lori and I agreed to tour Red Square and its surroundings, although I had reservations about this. I knew we stood out: Our La Sportiva trek boots matched, over the ankle with tan uppers and big black soles and heels. We contrasted with Lori having youthful shoulder length black hair while mine was a whitish gray. We both wore blue jeans. Even among other tourists, no one else looked like us. Because we didn't speak Russian, just navigating from place to place became a challenge.

Finding a train to downtown Moscow from the airport, where Red Square was located, seemed straightforward. We located signs in English and other languages and were soon on our way. This particular train made a continual out-and-back circuit from the airport to a drop off point, so we knew it would be available to take us back to the airport. Oh, that the second train was so easy.

Only a few passengers boarded the train, but they all shared a common trait with people in the busy bustling airport. I don't think a single person made eye contact with us, nor did anyone speak. While mildly disconcerting at first, this would soon become a problem for us.

At least the weather had a sunny disposition and temps were pleasant. We exited the first train after a slow, thirty minute ride to its terminus. Bowing to the tourists, signs in multiple languages pointed us to a subway station and further directions to the Red Square train.

Once we found the station and our second train, we were again engulfed by secondhand cigarette smoke. The second train was a subway and in Moscow these are far below street level. The interiors of the subway hallways were beautifully decorated with wall art.

"What's with the people?" Lori groused. "They aren't very nice, not friendly at all."

"Well, at least they're consistent," I added. "It's been like this since we got off the plane. Maybe we should get used to it. I expect this is how they treat tourists." Thinking quickly and to dispel future doubt, I added: "People in the mountains are more welcoming. Plus they're part of our team and working for us and with us—I'm sure it'll be different there." A prophet I am not, but I would be right about this, except for a gaffe caused by me.

After leaving the subway we boarded a long escalator that went up and up to reach street-level. Wistfully I thought, "This would be nice on the mountain!"

And then we stepped onto the street to find sunshine and people. Instantly we noticed both a marked difference, and similarities. Throngs of people milled about and they seemed friendly enough, but only to each other. Not to us. Downtown Moscow was lively in early summer, with young and middle aged people everywhere. The Russian women seemed tall and big, with high heels making them even taller. Some dressed fashionably, and almost all the women wore their hair styled and coifed, plus bracelets and other jewelry, high heels, and—cripes! The men all had cigarettes. People strolled around the square, smoking while enjoying the weather and each other.

Almost immediately in downtown Moscow we noticed a banner stretched across the roadway proclaiming in huge letters: "Welcome Wally Gomez."

I pointed to it and laughed. "Darn, they misspelled my last name." We never did find out who Wally Gomez was. Then an orange Lambourghini stopped almost directly in front of us. Still caught up in the banner, I said to Lori, "Looks like our limo is right on time."

I had purchased a Pontiac Solstice after returning from Everest, because my other vehicle (my beloved Aunt Angie's car from her estate) barely clung to life support. I began calling my new sports car a Lambourghini. So I got a kick when in Moscow the real thing pulled up and stopped almost right in front of us. The illusion ended in exhaust smoke when the traffic light changed. The car went one way and off we—cough—walked to Red Square through its exhaust smoke, which actually seemed milder than Moscow's pervasive cigarette exhaust.

Red Square was tour books and history books come alive. We saw the Kremlin, St. Basil's Cathedral with its colorful globe tipped spires, the huge GUM Department Store, and people dressed in period military costumes from the era of the Czar. We also saw armed soldiers on patrol.

The spectacular St. Basil's Cathedral especially caught my eyes, and we walked across Red Square toward its porticoes and bulbous colorful shapes. We were viewing an icon in person—breathtaking. As the government has tried to discourage and legislate religion, the Russians now call the church a state museum. Many other tourists were also viewing the cathedral.

A sideshow featured a small monkey on a short chain and an eagle on a perch, neither of them in cages. No one, including Lori and I, wanted to get close. Costumed characters included SpongeBob talking to person in a Spider Man costume. We lounged outside the Cathedral/museum and took selfies.

I probably disappointed Lori by deciding not to enter because I thought the fee was steep and I worried our funds might be tight. Again the prophet—more tight than I realized. However, I did find a few rubles for a begging woman who sat on the concrete in the open Square. I didn't hear anyone else speaking English. The languages around us sounded like Russian, some German, and Asian.

I didn't know the complete history of Russian power struggles across time, but I believed Red Square was the scene of many internal conflicts from the czars to present time. Thus, we stepped through a history of blood in this square.

Lori enjoyed shopping, so we helped the economy in Russia by entering the huge GUM department store, the world's biggest such enterprise under a single roof. This building was about the size of three connected soccer fields, standing three floors high and filled with retail shops and restaurants. The GUM site was a historic commerce center that originated along the banks of the nearby Minsk River where fishermen, trappers, and traders found mercantile opportunities as Moscow developed.

We did our part—Lori buying a T-shirt, and me ice cream cones for two. I don't know that we were in every shop, but if we missed seeing any it was only a few. Lori is a world class shopper, doing her thing in a world class venue.

Crowds of people thronged the eateries, shops, and subways. We noticed some litter, but no more than you'd expect in a large city. Downtown Moscow seemed fairly clean. Unfortunately, the people around us remained indifferent to our presence. No eye contact, no smiles. The Russian faces turned toward us looked dour and expressionless. Did they even see us? Between and among one another they expressed gaiety, especially the young people. But they treated us as invisible. Were we ugly Americans?

I had voiced caution about going downtown because I'm not always comfortable in urban areas, especially new ones. That was exacerbated by several factors. I told Lori, "Moscow has the potential to become a police state in a heartbeat. We don't speak the language. We can't read the weird Cyrillic character language. And, we don't know anyone."

Lori didn't disagree with me, but none of this made her timid or unsure. And, after all, she poured money into this trip, so the vacation belonged to her as much as me. Is climbing a mountain a vacation? Oh, hold that thought. Right now, thanks to Lori, we were shopping and sightseeing in downtown Moscow.

I did know a cousin attached to a Russian embassy, and we had communicated. While she said she'd be as helpful as possible if we had problems, she was on the other side of the country—and indeed Russia is a huge place. If things went south for whatever reason, especially in Moscow, we'd be in a world of hurt.

Generally, for me the glass is half full. I like to quote a Indy 500 driver Lyn St. James, from Aspen, Colorado, who said of her car owner, "If the glass only had a drop of water in it, he said it was half full." I heard her say that in person when she addressed a St. Vincent's leadership group. But I tempered her comment with realism, and Moscow was an appropriate place to be on alert. I wasn't anxious or worried; I was prepared.

Confusion reigned as we left Red Square. We retraced our steps to the metro area train station without difficulty, but my memory was fuzzy when it came to the correct subway line. This became a challenge of magnitude, because every escalator and departure point seemed identical. Subways went to all four Moscow airports, not just ours. The signs were confusing, at best.

After fifteen minutes seeking help from strangers, including police, we learned:

a) Some people in Russia will not respond to a request for help either because they don't speak your language or because they do speak your language, but just don't care to help; b) If you speak English, some people turn away immediately; c) The civil militia, the police, don't speak English as a rule. And, thankfully: d) Even in brusque and burly Russia, some kindly people were willing to help. Our rescuers were an older couple who, in halting English thick with Russian accents, directed us to the proper train and made certain we understood where to get off. Thank you, God, for them, and bless them.

We got to where we needed to be and, on our own, found our train back to the airport, the correct airport of the four. I blamed myself for the confusion. I thought I had memorized our route inbound to Red Square, but that wasn't the case. Still, nothing would be gained by beating myself up.

I pledged: *I must do better with details.*

In an airport pub we took our early evening dinner in the form of breakfast, eating Russian eggs washed down with German beer. Lori and I spoke of the day and of the next day, which would end at our mountain village. Meantime, our overnight plan was to sleep in "comfy" chairs at a coffee shop we patronized earlier. We also patronized it that night, buying cups of java, and lounging in the chairs, seeking sleep. We wouldn't fly out until first thing in the morning.

I suppose I should have seen it coming. When the coffee shop closed, we were evicted. I had noticed wooden benches at the far end of the terminal, so we hiked down there. Other people had the same idea, but thankfully a couple of benches remained vacant. The benches were about seven or eight feet long and shaped for sitting, not sleeping, so they were a little skinny for our bodies. Lori got one; I took another one. And thus, we found our overnight accommodations.

Sunday, June 20, 2010   Father's Day

Travel Day

The hard bench made for an uncomfortable, restless sleep, compounded by ceaseless and awful music from a closed bar across the airport corridor. Hoping to quiet my spirit, I thought about Father's Day, my son Dom, and my own deceased father. I hoped and prayed Dom and Kathryn and Siena were well and that the day would be special for Dom. I looked forward to extending this greeting to my other son Andy when he and Jill—God willing—became parents.

Talking to my deceased father is common to me. I tell my deceased close family members "Hello" on many mornings. Sometimes I say, "Thank you; I miss you; I love you." These messages keep the connection alive. Just because they're in heaven and I'm gravity-bound on Earth doesn't mean we can't communicate. Other times, I tell them my news and listen to hear if they have anything to say. For all they had to say on earth, (and I laugh as I consider this), they are mostly silent now.

In the morning I stirred awake on my bench bed, sore all over. Times two. Lori stirred also, feeling the same. We headed downstairs to retrieve our checked baggage. Our flight would depart from a gate upstairs. I secured a three wheeled luggage transport cart and struggled to fit everything on it. Tricky—and also heavy.

Our flight from Moscow went southwest across the vast countryside toward the Caucasus Mountains, where a future Olympics would be held just west of our destination, followed by Moscow military intervention and annexation. Our destination is considered one of the most deadly and rugged mountain ranges in the world. We were flying to a town called Mineral Vody, known for its springs. The flight took two hours and we were in a rickety plane that looked at least 50 years old. Talk about your caution alert warning system activating.

Thankfully, the alarm was not necessary. The crew and plane performed well. On schedule we landed at one of the smallest airports I had ever seen. And the Mineral Vody Airport restroom ranked as the second worst bathroom facility I had ever used. Scoring beneath Mineral Vody's airport john was the one in Kathmandu Airport in Nepal. The restroom smelled foul and looked worse than foul. Sanitation was unknown, suffice it to say. The things we Americans and the West take for granted is a theme that replays whenever I go on mountain expeditions.

The Mineral Vody Airport indoor restroom should have been closed by a board of health (and I wondered if such existed in Russia). Lori, an RN who hadn't been out of the USA was shocked. She'd never witnessed such a lack of hygiene although I warned her. In a couple of hours on our drive to the mountain this situation would go from airport bad, to convenience stop worse, at her first outdoor loo. On the mountain at our base camp it would be worse still. Well, at least I had prepared her for what to expect at base camp where outdoor toilets gave new meaning to the word *primitive*.

We collected our bags from the dirt and concrete floor. This airport had no fancy or even basic conveyor system. Despite what I saw and felt just now, after perils on and after the mountain, Lori and I would be delighted to return to this airport when we were finally able to travel home.

As we headed for the exit, consisting of a single set of double doors, I was struck by the poverty levels at the airport. Many people wore old, tattered, and torn clothing. Dental care was lacking. Luggage was as worn as the leathered faces of the people who unloaded our bags. Prayers for them. At home I would expect to see people begging. I did see beggars at Red Square and responded to them, but no begging here for some reason. I wondered about that.

Sergey, our expedition guide, was there to meet us and we also met James, originally from Ireland, who would make the climb with us. Sergey wore a bright blue jacket and was slim with his hair cropped close. He smiled little, and said less. What words of welcome he said were softly spoken in English accented by his native Russian tongue. He had not mastered English, and later I came to understand this, and that he knew it, and the deficit bothered him. He carried himself like a fit athlete.

James, who said we should call him Jim, lived in the states and worked as an international pilot for a package delivery company. He was as talkative and Sergey was silent. He wore dark colored clothing and had dark brown hair and a moustache. Stockier than most climbers I knew, he'd been a military pilot in England and—like me—had the Seven Summits in his sights.

The four of us boarded a minibus for a four hour drive from Mineral Vody, a city of natural springs, to a mountain village near Mount Elbrus called Terskol. Enroute we stopped for a sandwich and soda, plus a visit to the restroom. All the services at the stop were pricey. There was even a cost to use the loo. As I mentioned earlier, the loo left Lori, with her nursing and hospital background and absence of international travel, shall we say, alarmed. This primitive outdoor toilet hut was something people might've used in the United States during the last century.

As Lori discovered, the loos were all unsanitary and smelly, with no running water and usually no toilet paper. She hesitated to enter this, her first one, and quickly learned that, once inside, you must do your business, finish, and get out. Holding your breath and not looking about too much had benefits as well. The Russian locals had figured out they could charge for this convenience, located behind a kind of country store with a pop stand out front. Lori was appalled. Having been to Everest and Kilimanjaro, I knew this often was the norm and I wasn't surprised. Loos were not a part of our Indiana mountain training, although for urinary relief you grew accustomed to finding a spot when out in Hoosierland nature.

We visited with Jim as Sergey drove our bus along a two lane road to Terklot. We spotted the Caucasus range in the distance and soon the roadway began to rise and fall with the terrain. Here and there the narrow two lane road included a passing lane on our side, as we were driving uphill through mountainous terrain much of the way. Traffic was light. I recognized a few BMWs and Mercedes cars going to and from the mountain—I presumed they carried upscale skiers. For the most part, the vehicles I saw appeared to be Russian made, or imports I didn't recognize. Well, we did see the occasional VW.

In the next several days, this roadway from Terklot to Mineral Vody, normally a four hour drive, would become an embattled area, which represented the second mountain in Russia Lori and I would climb.

We had a nice hotel at Terklot, one of several in the small village about ten miles from the trailhead to Elbrus. Terklot was also a gateway to skiing which continued even during the summer, because Elbrus is made up of glaciers and permanent snowfields.

So while the calendar said June, people still rode the lifts to ski down the mountain on its lower reaches where they enjoyed warmer temps. The most stalwart skiers would take off their skis and hike higher up the mountain for a more out-of-bounds back-country skiing experience. Some of these people paid extra and rode upward in a motor-power and tread-equipped people-carrier called a snow cat. Depending on how these so-called snow cats are fabricated, one can ride inside or outside.

I was exhausted on checking-in and grabbed a few winks of sleep before dinner. Lori was exhausted too, except she missed dinner and slept around the clock. Travelling halfway around the world is stressful for both mind and body.

Monday, June 21, 2010

First Day of Summer

My back pack contained my smallish Bible and I spent some time reading after awakening about 5 a.m. Russian time. The time differential between home and Moscow was big, with Moscow nine hours ahead. Jet lag, plus the variance, threw us off balance— Lori a little more than me. She awakened later and we headed down to the hotel restaurant for breakfast. A meal plan was part of our program: The See Food Diet, meaning I would eat almost whatever I saw. Lori was especially hungry, having not eaten the night before. I chowed down on porridge, dried fruit, raw fruit, dark Russian bread which I absolutely loved, hot tea, two big sunny side up eggs, and orange juice.

We visited with Jim at breakfast. I had dinner with him the night of our arrival and found him delightful, although talkative to the point of monologue. I say this with non-judgment as I share this gift—or is it a curse? The same waitress from the previous night, young, thin, and with a beautiful smile, waited on us this morning.

Unlike people at the airport, she was nicely dressed, clean, and her dental work was in order. She seemed a bit shy.

We met Sergey in the hotel lobby and it was time to get started. Off we trekked for 20 minutes to Alps Industria, our outfitter, to get our trek poles. We would get our other gear later. We each had backpacks and water, having been told by Sergey to expect an acclimatizing hike that would take much of the day. Seregy wasn't what I'd call unfriendly; he was, well, Russian. He just didn't say a lot; He made eye contact while speaking to us, but he was never an idle talker. Economy of language I called this. As I got to know him and realized his second language of English tripped him up, I grasped he felt self-conscious and possibly a bit shy. I would find on the mountain that, when necessary, he knew how to be direct. As he got to know us, Sergey loosened up and could even laugh.

Off we trekked for another 30 minutes to a ski lift where we would catch a ride into the steeper glaciated terrain. Today's morning and early afternoon workout provided an opportunity to acclimatize to the elevation, plus give us a good climb. It would also allow Sergey to asses our mountaineering skills. The climb took us to a mountain in Elbrus' shadow, (well it would have been in the shadow if the sun were shining). We were in a range of mountains that offered snow skiing, but on this day we would not see skiers or other climbers.

We arrived before the lift opened and the operator hadn't arrived. I found this a hoot because it reminded me of numerous mornings when I showed up early at ski lifts from Chile, to British Columbia, to Colorado, to West Virginia, to Indiana (yes, we do have a ski resort in southern Indiana). My eagerness to get first tracks on the mountain was a benchmark of many years of skiing. This meant I wished to be among the first skiers to board the lift, if not *the* first. Being first in line translates to being first down the mountain—hence "first tracks." Sometimes I'd show up before the ski lift operators arrived. No different on this day, although we were a long way from home.

Hold the phone. Something seemed different on this lift. As Lori and I, Jim, and Sergey waited, up walked eight men dressed in military uniforms, carrying weapons the likes of which I never saw in my Army days. They appeared to be automatic rifles, with short stocks. Were the stocks plastic? I have eight years of military background and spent time in foreign countries, but never in Russia. Jim also had a military background from England, but he didn't recognize the weapons either. We also didn't recognize the insignia. Were they Russian border guards for the Elbrus territory, or not? They stayed off to the side away from us. Unlike us, they were there on business. Like us, they waited.

Mount Elbrus, the highest summit in Russia, counts as the highest summit in continental Europe. Russia is considered part of the European continent. Elbrus's geography and military history make interesting reading, past and present. Its location and the present political climate made it too interesting, as Lori and I would soon discover.

Hitler's Germany invaded Russia during World War II. One Nazi break-through across the Russian border came right where we were. Millions of lives were lost as Hitler's invasion gained ground, with his forces over-powering Stalin's Red Army. Led by tanks, the German Army stream-rolled across Russia toward Moscow. Some military historians believe the loss of life on both sides and its significance in the war equaled or even surpassed the United States' atomic bombing of Hiroshima and Nagasaki, Japan.

The Elbrus Territory, where we were, borders Georgia, which has a rich reserve of oil fields, some of the largest in the world. As Germany depleted its own oil supply on which the tanks and transportation of the war effort depended, oil was sought from other countries. The oil-rich deposits in Chechnya, Baku, and Grozny were in Georgia. Georgia was to our immediate south. From the high flanks of Elbrus we could see over the Caucasus into Georgia.

Hilter's military invasion into this region was code-named Operation Barbarosa. Hitler's invasion of Russia in 1941, began on June 22, exactly 69 years ago (minus one day) from that day in Elbrus. Our lives had intersected both history and geography. In a couple of days I almost held in my hands a newly discovered and definitive artifact of that history and geography.

With Georgia and its oil lying just south of Mount Elbrus, and Georgia being just north of Iraq and Iran, Chechnya was described to me as "a powder keg," by a former Department of State diplomat who would know.

As I looked at our armed and uniformed ski lift neighbors, I wondered if this squad of soldiers were border guards reporting to duty somewhere on the mountain where the military had a frontier encampment. Maybe... maybe not. I certainly didn't care to ask them.

I considered all this as we rode up the lift, which finally opened. The military men and their firepower took the first chairs. That was fine by me even though we arrived earlier. No first tracks today anyway. We boarded the lift next.

If you've been on an American ski lift, say a four person quad chair in Colorado, where an attendant helps passengers board, figure our Elbrus lift was on the other end of the spectrum. Each lift chair seated only one person, and the chairs on the lift were unattended for boarding. The lift operator was by himself at his control panel inside a nearby hut. The lift continually moved until he stopped it.

We were boarding with back packs, which could be tricky. And Lori had never been on a ski lift. Geez oh Pete. Thankfully, the operator must have sensed me hovering about as her chair neared and he came out and helped her board safely, controlling the chair's swinging movement. "Thank you," I said in English. If he said anything I missed it.

I felt comfortable boarding solo, but the back pack made me a little unstable. Again, he steadied the chair. "Thanks again."

Silence. Sergay and Jim were already on their way. It started to rain lightly as we went up. I expected the rain would change to snow as we moved higher.

We all wore warm mountaineering clothing that provided the dry warmth we'd need today. Our objective was to ascend 1,700 feet of elevation, up to 12,000 feet was my understanding. The climbing aspect, or angle of the slope, was 35 to 40 degrees in some places, Jim said. I wondered about that, since we wouldn't be roping up. Roping up is when each of us ties into a rope and the rope is connected to at least one other climber for safety reasons.

The boulders we encountered that day, big and small, were challenging to me, not to mention Lori. Some smaller boulders were snow covered with maybe their top halves or thirds protruding above the snow line. Larger ones protruded completely out of the snow. Their location was not aligned with the fall line we ascended to gain elevation, but Sergey directed us to climb a number of different boulders so he could assess our abilities. These boulders were longer rather than taller. So we practiced climbing up onto them, traversing across them, then dismounting, and repeating the process in the boulder field.

Coaching from Sergey and Jim was helpful on this terrain. The rocks were wet and slippery from the rain and snowmelt, and icy slick in spots. From today's clouds, the moisture continued as drizzle. The slopes weren't as steep as advertised—yet. I had not done a lot of this bouldering on previous climbs and Lori had done none. We found this experience helpful, though challenging.

As we gained altitude, previous snows had buried the rocks. Now the air temperature was cold enough to consolidate the snow texture. We would climb on top of the snow until it broke through here and there and we sank up to our knees. But the going remained fairly stable. The rain stopped and sunlight teased us, peeking out for a few minutes at a time. Clouds returned, but no more rain or snowfall, for the moment. We climbed up and up and up, with the slope getting steeper, yet manageable. We were without crampons, but if the slope was any steeper or icier they'd have been a must.

Up and up and up. Uh,oh. I spotted a huge cornice above us to the left, resembling a wave frozen in relief. I was concerned it could slab—break free and fall. As in fall toward us. To my relief, Sergay detoured us around it. Thank you very much, Sergey. Thank you, God that this wave didn't break. That mother was huge.

Finally we gained the summit at about 12,000 feet in elevation. As the clouds cleared a bit, we saw breathtaking views in all directions. We stopped on a comfortable saddle, taking time to appreciate where we were and how we got there. We hydrated and ate. I said a quick "Thank you" to God, expressing gratitude for our bodies, minds, and spirits. The time was 1:34 p.m. in Russia—time for lunch on the mountain. The Indiana lunch rest spots where Lori and I ate while climbing looked way different than this. At Brown County State Park near the Fire Tower we reached about 1,000 feet elevation. Said another way, that was 11,000 feet below where we perched and half a world away around the globe. Just the same, Brown County was good to us as a training site. Mill Race Park in Columbus with its observation tower (Thanks to the Force and Shumaker families) and earthen mound on the back side of the Mill Race Amphitheater were helpful also.

The sack lunch Sergey provided contained a big green juicy apple, a hardboiled egg, some kind of pressed sausage on that delicious dark bread I loved, a layered crispy chocolate something or other, and a candy bar. I ate everything but the candy bar. Lori did likewise except for the sausage—no beef or pork products for this diet-conscious woman. Lori and I reminded each other to hydrate, hydrate, hydrate. This mantra would get more interesting on our Elbrus summit day.

Today we saw mountains in all directions. As this was a ski area and not far from the site of where the 2014 Winter Olympics would be held, we saw many runs, a lift here and lodges there. But all that was down, down toward the valley. Up where we were, with the tricky terrain and no lift access, only serious, even elite, out of bounds skiers would venture. The only way to reach these areas, presuming you wanted to, was to remove your skis, shoulder them, and hike up. I suppose ski cats as tracked winter ATVs might make it here, but we saw no sign of tracks or skiers.

Excitement followed lunch as we began our descent at the top of a long and steep snow slope, one of the steepest seen on that day. Our climbing partner Jim made a misstep, lost his balance, and fell. He began sliding feet first down the mountain. He was uphill from me, and his slide headed my way. He artfully veered around me and then tumbled forward as his slide continued. I expect he traveled 50 yards down mountain before he could bring himself to a stop. As we watched Jim, Lori suddenly fell also, and her slide brought her into direct contact with me. I felt like head pin in a bowling alley. She knocked me over, and down we went. Fortunately I got the both of us stopped before we traveled far. About then Jim shouted he was okay.

Sergey came over to Lori and I and demonstrated how to use trek poles to put on the brakes during a fall. In mountaineering this is called self-arrest. Probably he should have covered this in advance, I told myself. Sergey would later cover self-arrest during our ice axe training. Guess he didn't see this coming.

I thought about this trek pole self-arrest teaching as we covered the steep distance down to where Jim waited. Sergey had Lori in hand, holding her backpack straps. He slowly eased her down the mountain as she slid on her behind. Game to use the teaching just learned, I begin an intentional slow glissade down the mountain. In control, this was fun. Raise up your feet and lay back with trek poles pulled up you gain speed. To dump speed you drag the trek poles and begin using your feet as brakes. It worked pretty well. I would pick up speed, arrest, speed up, slow down. I was having fun with this because it reminded me of descending a mountain on skis.

A sharp whistle from Sergey brought me to a halt. I heard a second sharp whistle. When I looked around, I was down mountain a fair ways from them. Sergey was signaling me to cross the mountain horizontally to intersect their diagonal downward direction. Good thing I stopped when I did. Much farther and I would have had an uphill climb to re-group.

On our summit day I would hear Sergey's whistle again. It remains the most memorable whistle of my life.

Jim sustained a forehead cut and knot from his tumble and grumbled some. I thought better of saying anything.

We continued our descent with no more falls. After a fair hike we came round a hill and spotted the high point turn-around terminus for another rickety looking lift. Lori was a little way ahead of me. This was another single chair like before, and this time the attendant didn't even bother coming out of his little shack to attend the chair. Lori started boarding the chair. Uh, oh! She was unaccustomed to ski lifts, so I had to yell at her to direct her attention to the approaching chair. She got distracted and didn't see the next chair coming. I waved her off. On getting there I told her, a little heatedly, that even with my years of experience with ski lifts these single chairs were skittish. "This is no time for an injury. Let me help you board these things. Please," I said.

Lori proved herself strong on the climb, but her fall and the lift chair incident prompted concern in me about her inexperience in a mountain environment. Those thoughts occupied my mind as the lift carried us down. Eventually I began noticing the beautiful scenery of verdant hills and stands of green pines at this lower elevation. I smelled fireplace fires from the ski cabins. I reminded myself I had always wanted to summer ski, and here I was faux skiing—sledding down a mountain on my bottom on the very day of summer solstice. I had skied in the Andes in Chile a couple of Septembers, which was spring in the Southern Hemisphere. But today was summer in the northern hemisphere, the one I lived in. My "skiing" in the Caucasus Mountains didn't involve boards on my feet, but my imagination had fun with the notion.

We trekked into the village to our outfitter, Alps Industria, to pick up the rest of our gear. There we met, for the first time, Victoria, our official Russia expedition sponsor representing the outfitter. My understanding was all foreign Elbrus visitors, especially Americans, had sponsors. What today was business as usual with an intermediary would later become vitally important to us. There were some negotiations over credits and allowances concerning equipment rental. That completed, Victoria presented us with Elbrus Summit T-shirts even though we hadn't set foot on the mountain.

I really don't like receiving the shirts in advance. This reminded me of Everest and securing T-shirts proclaiming in advance my climb to the top of 18,200 elevation Kala Patar, in connection with our trek to Everest Base Camp at 17,600. I bought the T-shirts for both Base Camp and Kala Patar when I found a good deal. The problem was, I hadn't yet climbed Kala Patar and for good reason I ended up passing on it. Not having climbed Kala Patar, I actually returned the T-shirts to the store for a refund. My hubris buying them in advance cost me—in humility. And it cost me practically too as I got less than half my money back on exchange, despite my protest.

It didn't help today when Jim wryly observed about the T-shirts, "You have to give it back if you don't summit." However, as they were the last shirts in stock, we took them, not wanting our "gold medals" to land on the backs of other climbers. Lori, however, did object to being issued the incorrect size. She stayed the course and somehow persuaded them to find her correct size despite the shelves being empty. Well, good for her. The outfitter's van delivered us to our hotel. I doubled the driver's tip as I had stiffed him on the ride from the airport, not having correct denominations. I apologized, noting the increase. The man didn't speak English, but he did understand rubles. He smiled and vigorously shook my hand.

Jim joined Lori and I for dinner. His conversation skills made for an interesting and lengthy meal, because he told good stories with lots of detail. Then it was time to head to our room for important work. We packed and repacked our backpacks, taking only essentials needed for the climb. The next morning after breakfast we would check out of the hotel and head up to our Elbrus base camp, called The Barrels.

I fell asleep early and slept through the night except for pee bottle breaks, although for now in the hotel we had the convenience of a bathroom. I looked out the window and saw stars galore.

Tuesday, June 22, 2010

Birdsong was my alarm about 5 o'clock in the morning, just like in Indiana. Not sure what species of birds I heard, but they carried a beautiful tune. God gifts us with an absolutely gorgeous dawn rung in by the birds...Thank you, Elohim Creator God. I read some Psalms based in nature from my mini Bible and said prayers for safety. I missed my family, although Lori was excellent company. It wasn't the same as family or my guy friends who would do something like this, but nice to have someone from home along. Well, what guy friends did I have, God love them all, who would do this? I laughed. They were much too smart—just ask them! Anyway, at Everest and Kilimanjaro I was on the expedition with crews, none of whom I knew until we all arrived. I welcomed the diversity in the make-up of climbers and the guides.

Here and now, I had someone along for the adventure who came from Indiana, from my culture and my organization, and was involved in leading the work my treks supported. Lori was good company, she was game, and her strength equaled her enthusiasm although her inexperience in the mountains was as vast as the mountains themselves.

In the dining room, we feasted on a large breakfast, and my plate included a little of everything. Was there something different about those eggs this morning? They seemed a bit suspicious, but I ate them. Next we headed down to the hotel basement with the luggage we would leave behind. We jammed all that gear into a couple of tall, narrow lockers set aside by the hotel for skiers and climbers to use. The lockers were good-size, and so was our gear. It was a tight squeeze, but finally we shoehorned everything inside. Then, Lori, myself, and Jim were to meet Sergay in the lobby with the van driver. After loading the van, we headed toward the mountain's base.

Our excitement was building.

We each loaded our backpacks with what we'd need for the climb, which would be a considerably shorter duration than Everest and Kilimanjaro. Those expeditions were ten to fourteen days on the mountains. In contrast, we would only spend about 14 days total in Russia. Mount Elbrus would essentially be a one-day (one very long day), climb. However, we needed training and acclimatizing to make the climb safe, and even possible.

The previous day was step one, as we ascended about 2,000 feet up the neighboring mountain to 12,000 elevation and began acclimatizing. We still had techniques to learn with ice axe self-arrest, climbing in mountaineering boots with crampons attached, and glacier travel up and down a mountain. We would also learn about climbing while tied into a rope. These days of crucial training aimed to ensure our long summit day climb would be safe and, hopefully, successful. Meanwhile, our remarkable human bodies would acclimatize during the training conducted at elevation.

We arrived at the Elbrus ski village base after a ten mile drive. On our approach, the twin peaks of Elbrus came into view. Oh, my—gulp! We viewed the peaks from a distance on this beautiful day. They looked magnificent and tall, two clean and somewhat squat white pyramids towering above the countryside.

We boarded a tram ski lift to gain a few hundred feet, and the peaks became foreshortened as we approached them more closely on the lift. On this sunny morning, many skiers also boarded the tram. And here we came without skis. Instead we toted backpacks and 40 gallon blue mountaineering barrels filled with food and climbing gear, such as ropes and safety gear.

We met Leanne, who would serve as our happy chef, keeping us well fed. She also nourished me with her big bear hugs. Contrary to the Russian disposition we came to expect, Leanne carried some joy within her. She wasn't bubbly and over-talkative, but had a natural smile that came easily. I presumed her to be from a nearby mountain village as she radiated the kind of warmth most mountain people the world over seem to have. As with many cooks, her girth suggested she enjoyed the food she prepared. She was Lori's height and wore a warm, puffy Alps Industria logoed jacket and mountaineering pants. Strong, she easily toted one of the blue barrels that contained our food stores. Lori loved nutrition and cooking, and as the two women in our party of five, they had lots to talk about. Like Sergey, Leanne wasn't fluent in English, but she was more willing to try.

We all toted our own gear plus the community barrels up the ski tram's flights of stairs and onto the tram cabs. We took the first tram, rode up and arrived, unloaded gear, and then reloaded it onto a second tram to get closer to our base camp. With some envy, I watched skiers and snowboarders flash down the mountain. The first lift hovered above the lovely Ukraine hill country. The second tram lifted us high into the Edelweiss summer of the glaciated mountain known as Elbrus.

Beneath us, skiers and snow boarders came alive in the glory of speedy descents. I enjoyed watching their late morning warm weather turns. Warmer temps from the sun soften the overnight frozen snow, turning it into manageable "corn," as skiers call the hero snow that is easy to carve turns through. Early morning frozen snow is a little more challenging to negotiate. However, late in the afternoon the goddess of corn snow goes rogue bitchy when it gets too soft and the soupiness makes a mess of the mountains.

When we reached the end of the second lift, the bluebird sky scenery became more interesting, as we could see more and more above and below us. Elbrus' twin peaks, one just higher than the other, edged up beyond the crowns of their neighbors. They were resplendent white cones thrust into a cloudless blue sky. Did I whisper a prayer that our summit day weather would look like this? Finally, we boarded a snow cat that would move us toward our base camp on Elbrus.

Some purists might say, "Well you didn't climb the mountain all the way, now did you?" While it's true we didn't climb the portion where we were lifted by mechanized means, we did ascend 2,000 feet the day before during the acclimatizing hike. During additional training in the next few days we would go well over the distance we ascended with motorized help.

The same principle is true today of the elite women and men who climb Everest. They get a head start flying in choppers or fixed wing aircraft from Kathmandu to Lukla, covering many linear miles and a few thousand feet, just as I did on my trek to Everest Base Camp by taking the same flight. Who am I to tell them, they didn't climb the whole route? While training, the first summiteers of Everest climbed vertically up and down three times the height of the mountain before making their summit attempt. This is part of acclimatizing.

We deposited our gear at our mountain home called The Barrels. The first thing to say is that the three of us, Lori, myself, and Jim were in Barrel Seven. For me this was a gift, as I consider seven a divine number going back to Genesis and the Creation story of six days of creation and God resting on day seven.

I am not a fundamentalist who says God created the world in precisely measured human time of seven days with 24 hours each. Such is possible certainly if God wished to do it that way, and perhaps He did. He can fully educate me about that when (hopefully) I reach Heaven. But I bow to science and accept that seven days on the clock we keep did not exist for the ancients, nor is it God's time. His sense of time is timeless. The Greek word kairos describes how God keeps time—divinely and timelessly. The Greek word chronos is how man keeps time with clocks and calendars.

These mountains evolved over hundreds of thousands of years—and they are still geo-physically changing. Further, I think that within the Bible, poetry, rhyme, metaphor and mystery co-exist. Here and now while I trek and climb this amazing planet, I don't require black and white scientific answers to all my questions, including those about creation. Should we not be careful about expecting the Bible to instruct us in science? That was never its purpose.

All these thoughts would percolate in my head during the next few days in Barrel 7. I felt we'd been given a sacred address on this mountain—thank You so much.

Practically speaking, the barrels were unused underground petroleum storage tanks converted to Spartan living quarters. Said another way, in America you'd pump your gas from one of these. Who gets to say they stayed in such a place? After we squared away our gear it was time for a quick lunch, then another training climb on this sunny, glorious day to be alive and in the mountains with fullness of body-mind-spirit. Such a gift. Off we went—Sergay, Jim, Lori, and me.

Uh,oh. Shortly into the training climb something felt amiss inside me. Surely not. My GI tract was tying itself into knots. We were some ways now from The Barrels, outfitted in climbing gear, back packs on, trek poles in our hands, and heading upward. The intestinal discomfort threatened to become a leak. I would need to make a pit stop soon—as in immediately!

Fortunately, a mechanized snow cat was parked not far away and I saw it as a men's room. Sergey was out in front, Jim second, Lori just ahead of me, and seemingly no one else nearby. I used the snow cat for support leaning against one of its huge treads to do what comes naturally from diarrhea. This was so embarrassing. Yes, I was indisposed. But the good news was, I had no fever or nausea. Thank you, God as this could have been so much worse. So I went. And went. And then I resumed the trek with only a few minutes lost. I had called to Lori to advise her of what was, well, coming down. She hung back to wait, and then I picked up the pace to rejoin Sergey and Jim. As if on cue, our sunny day soured into cloudy grayness seemingly commiserating with my malaise.

My GI scenario grew worse as the diarrhea occurred three more times. Seldom is the big D of diarrhea complete without multiple episodes. And that was annoying, but thankfully did not weaken me. Sergey and our group continued trekking upward. Sergay, to whom I confessed my problem, got annoyed with me at one of my pit stops. This wasn't because I was slowing us down, but because he was embarrassed for what others might see.

"Walter, Go over there behind the rocks" he said, indicating a rock island a quarter mile away.

"Sergey, if I could get there I would," was my first point to him. Second point: "As I have to go now, this place will do. And, if I offend you," I said, getting to what I think is the point as no else is around, "Then look the other way."

I preserved my dignity. He shut up. I leaned against a marker pole on the trail. And, oh I felt so much better. Hopefully that would be the end of it. I stayed absolutely calm through all of this, including when I got snowed on in a change of the weather. "Dump for a dump" I told myself with a smile.

We Catholics pray to many saints who carry prayers to God, but a gastro-intestinal tract saint is not one I know of. So I prayed directly to God, who in human form—complete with a GI tract—came to earth as enfleshed Jesus. I send my prayer request: "Jesus, I need some help here, please. Now. Thank you."

I mostly kept up with the group. After each pit stop I tried to tidy up the area so no one would know. In my mountaineering future I would learn from Rainier Mountaineering Inc. about blue, biodegradable human waste collection bags for these circumstances and nature calls. But that would be for other mountains. At this time and place, like a cat, I covered the mess as best I could.

Today we would ascend again about 2,000 feet, this time to about 13,000 feet elevation. We gained all 2,000 feet, about half a mile of vertical climbing, by steadily placing one foot in front of another . . . one foot in front of another . . . one foot in front of another.

This day became a kind of Judgment Day. Let me explain: Lori had never been to a Seven Summits mountain. In fact, she'd only been on one mountain—Pikes Peak, a 14,000 footer in Colorado. That was her mountain climbing resume before we came to Russia.

The good news was her high level of fitness. However, emotional preparation would become an issue, along with other fundamental facets of the mountain. The thin air of elevation required acclimatization. Crampons and an ice axe were new to her, as they were for me. Neither of us had tied in to a rope. So we both had things to learn, but I was fortunate that this was my third of the Seven Summits in three years. However, the learning curve for Lori would be as steep and formidable as Mount Elbrus' aspect, or slope angle. She felt confident the learning was within her grasp.

This was no surprise to either of us. I hoped I hadn't let her enthusiasm blur my judgment.

As a part of my learning curve, I found to my dismay, that Serey would be our only guide. He had no plans for a backup or auxiliary guide. This was dumb, and I said so. Jim and I viewed this differently. Unlike Lori, Jim had climbed some of the Seven Summits and intended to climb all of them. He was experienced. Resolving the guide issue would involve some tension between us.

All these issues became hues that colored this day—a day for celebration when Lori would mark a PR, personal record, for elevation. That was indeed good news.

But something else colored the day. As we down climbed, Lori's strides and speed caused her to pull away from me. Quickly she pulled ahead and got out of ear shot to my calls of "Poley poley!" A Swahili expression I learned at Kilimanjaro, it translates to "Slowly, slowly." This is the admonition African guides use to help ambitious climbers avoid mountain sickness from rushing up Kilimanjaro. I taught this principle to Lori at our Brown county training sessions as her gait allowed her to pull ahead of me. Well now she was way ahead. And, darn it, she didn't have the good sense to look back and see where I was. This wasn't about discourtesy, it was a judgment lapse. I was hopping mad about this. I thought: "She needs to think and act clearly."

In fairness, she was open with me about having some attention issues. But we could afford none of those deficits now. Sergey and Jim were a ways ahead of her and she was following their lead. But she wasn't cognizant that I was steadily falling farther behind. She needed to check her blind side, her back side. Finally after 35 to 40 minutes of her being out in front without checking to see where in heck I might be as she followed Sergey, Lori stopped. Our paths had diverged some around a rock outcropping, and near where she paused our two paths reunited, actually and metaphorically as it turned out. We resumed trekking together and she didn't say much.

I was steamed, but wished to remain calm. I often asked people I pastorally counseled: "What does calmness beget?"

Very few know the correct answer: "Calmness."

I didn't want to fly into a temper tantrum. I simply said, "Hey, I got a question for you?" I pointed out what had happened for the last 35 to 40 minutes and asked Lori directly: "Do you think I would have done that to you? And by that, I mean would I gone off and left you without looking back to check and see where you were and how you were doing?' I didn't wait for an answer. I made clear how we shared responsibility for safety.

"That means we watch out for not only ourselves, but for each other. There are significant safety aspects to consider on this mountain, and you just went on walkabout like this is Brown County State Park's paved roadways," I said firmly.

She paused and considered my words and tone. Then Lori apologized. This was caused by Lori's inexperience and naïvete, and worse—it was careless and sloppy behavior. This was no time to be distracted. We had covered such safety aspects during Indiana training. Like I said, this was a judgment day.

I also realized more judgment needed to follow about a backup guide—and the next step would be taking the lead for a discussion with Jim.

More acclimatizing work, communication, coordination, and training would help Lori and I work together better to deal with the mountain issues. However, Lori's mountain seasoning would also come by way of emotional preparation—amid a crisis of confidence the afternoon before our summit day.

The day's training trek ended and we arrived back at The Barrels base camp. My first priority was getting with Jim to have a frank, hopefully short, discussion about the backup guide. I was adamant that safety demanded we have an auxiliary guide. He disagreed, but he did listen. We were both tired and agreed maybe some rest would do us both good and we'd take a run at the idea after sleeping.

The tiny window in Barrel 7 faced west, and Lori and I had bunks on the west end on either side of the room. The window was set above a table in the middle, with a beautiful alpenglow sunset streaming into the room. Jim slept in the front end of The

Barrel, near the only door access to our quarters. No OSHA or ADA requirements for alternate exits on a Russian mountain when sleeping inside a petroleum can.

I was exhausted and fell to sleep quickly. Lori awakened me later, saying I was snoring.

Wednesday, June 23, 2010

I visited the loo early in the morning, feeling secondary cramps in my GI tract. No one was awake, so I lay in bed and I followed my practice of naming God using names and titles from Scripture—I got to 115 by the time Lori began to stir ten feet across the room, and soon Jim awakened, about 20 feet away from us in his area. The naming of God and my time in the loo were the only peace I would get for a while.

Jim came to our doorway and Lori asked, "How did you sleep?" Wrong question. Jim began to stridently rant about my snoring, saying I kept him awake and that he needed his sleep. My snoring, he said, robbed him of that sleep. The rest of this day went downhill from there.

There are no two ways about saying this: Jim was plenty pissed. At me. His attitude did not improve when (in his opinion) I became defensive in a smart aleck way. Jim found my come-back comments "unacceptable." Oh, boy—my big mouth.

I said something about "my snores covering all the notes of a ten piece orchestra" or something stupid like that, making light of a matter he considered serious. He didn't say he found that unfunny or condescending or disrespectful, but his actions the rest of the day made it clear that, along with the snoring, my attitude was way in the wrong.

When we were alone I tried to atone for the snoring and inane remarks with an apology. I offered words of reconciliation. He would have none of it. And so a deep quiet began between the two of us. His last words to me for several hours were: "We just need to focus."

Well, I wished those were his last words. Another verbal fusillade followed about the snoring and the capricious remark I made.

My choice was to let it go. I had sincerely apologized. I could do no more. Lori and I received total silence and disassociation the likes of which I had never personally experienced. During the day's training, at breaks on the mountain, he purposefully sat away from Lori and I with his back turned.

I told myself, "It isn't my problem now. He can carry this for as long as he wishes. I can do no more. He's the one who needs to budge, if he cares to." I realized his attitude could make for a long trip—especially because at some point we would all be roped together climbing one of the Seven Summits.

In order to function, I told myself: "Take a deep breath. Get yourself centered. Compartmentalize. This is now, today. Roping up will be then, and that, after all is for the future. Don't get ahead of yourself. Say some prayers Walter, why don't you? And leave it alone." So I did say prayers.

Obviously, this was not a good time to further discuss the open issue of the second guide. Tactically, I could wait; we still had time.

Elbrus, today, was another matter. What a glorious day for climbing. "Thank you, God for my body, mind, and spirit. Thank you for this beautiful, rugged environment. Help us be safe on a mountain I know can suddenly and unpredictably turn violent and dangerous with its perilous weather changes. Today, however, God through Mother Nature, You have gifted us with a calm day with sun, some clouds, and a light breeze. The climbing conditions are ideal. Thanks so much."

We strapped our crampons on for about a 1,200 foot elevation gain and the ascent went well for Lori and for me. We had worn these same crampons at home to train on the earthen mound at Mill Race Park and get a feel for going up and down in them. The mound was perhaps 45 feet high with a gentle brow to it, perfectly suited for growing accustomed to crampon-stepping.

I had increased my use and versatility for the crampons. I'd strap them onto my boots every time I mowed my yard. I'd slip my back pack on as well to simulate this 18,500 glaciated mountain even though I was in Indiana at 600 feet of elevation walking on grass. My neighbors stifled their guffaws as best they could. I know I made for a sight. Thankfully, no one in white coats showed up to take me away.

When we first strapped on the crampons on the mountain, grass and dirt still clung to the tines (24 steel points) of each set of our crampons. I told Lori we were leaving our mark on Russian territory by depositing Hoosier soil.

We tightened the crampon straps securely to our boots. When we walked and climbed, points bit into the snow, letting the teeth provide the stable footing mountaineers call "purchase." Our crampons worked satisfactorily and we performed well in them. The training at home had helped. Mowing your yard in crampons— you read it first here!

On this training day we steadily climbed up and up on a mountain climbing trail that ran parallel to a ski run. No ski lifts came this high, but snow cats hauled people to this elevated area. Perhaps a few stalwart souls took off their skis, put them across their shoulders, and hiked up. Having done that often at Aspen resorts, I could relate.

I thought how awesome the skiers' descent would be: 4,000-plus feet down to The Barrels where there was a lift. Or, they could ski farther down. I didn't know the exact descent, but the village was at least another 2,000 feet down the mountain. What a rock and roll ski journey that would be—6,000 feet and more. And this was summer skiing, something I longed to do.

Lori and I congo'd up the mountain behind Sergey. Further behind came Jim, still sulking. As we walked I mused about the ski lifts—the rickety ones, the larger trams, and the ski cats to get people up the mountain. This time we followed that route one step at a time, not parking our butts on a lift as I had done on 33 consecutive years of skiing in the American West. Here on Elbrus we climbed. Yet, many Russians enjoyed the mountain in a more conventional way. Like Americans, they would board a lift, go up, and let gravity suck them down the mountain as fast as they wanted to go. Good for them. When my climbing body ached, I envied them as we toiled upward, and then back down, one step at a time.

My thought process was interrupted as a guy skied up to us and, with a sliding stop, playfully sent a wave of snow our way. He called enthusiastically to Lori, "Ah, my American friend!" And they visited. Who was this? I wondered. After a few moments, Lori introduced me to the guy as her climbing partner and I recognize a man she met at the Alps Industria retail store when we rented our climbing gear. And from that brief encounter he recognized her. No surprise—she is an attractive and memorable woman.

Throughout this day today, Lori stayed mindful of me and my progress on the mountain and we stayed in communication. Our time together was coordinated. Yesterday's lesson was learned.

I felt more fatigue than I expected as we descended, which concerned me. On Kilimanjaro my fatigue when descending from the summit slowed me down. I don't want a re-occurrence of that.

We did have an arduous climb that day. If my math was correct we ascended 4,400 feet up from The Barrels, from 11,300 to 15,700 of elevation. My Go Zone Virgin Health Miles pedometer recorded

15,862 steps for the roundtrip, all of up and then down, kind of like our relationship with Jim.

As we arrived back at The Barrels we ran into another expedition group, plus in the distance we noticed a couple of people who appeared to be by themselves on the mountain. These latter two caught my attention. As they neared us, I saw one of them carrying an odd-looking trek pole. When he drew closer I wondered if my eyes were playing tricks on me. He was using a rifle as a trek pole, an ancient looking gun with a bayonet fixed to the rifle barrel. The stock was a single, long wooden piece, attached to a long barrel with a bolt action. This was an antique by today's standards, especially in view of the weapons we saw the border guards carrying. I expect it was 50 years old at least. From conversation in Russian and translation, we learned these guys had found the rifle that day, not far from where we stood. It lay frozen beneath the snow and ice for who knows how long, but seemed to be in excellent condition.

The finder man spoke Russian, fast and loud, as he showed off this rifle. Translated by Sergey, he told a remarkable story of finding the rifle on a kind of seam in the glacier.

While examining his find, I remembered this day was the anniversary of Germany's invasion of Russia. And here this guy found a rifle that looked to be World War II vintage.

As the owner of rifles, and having an interest in military history and some interest in its antiquities, I gestured a wish to hold the rifle. The man's monologue went silent and his face closed like an iron curtain. He pulled the gun close to his body and put his other arm out toward me as though to warn me off. He wasn't about to part with his find, if only for a minute to let a stranger hold it, especially one who spoke English.

Earlier, Jim had characterized the resolute standoffishness of the Russian people as though "you are trying to take something from them." I disagreed with his characterization until now. The man's gesture reflected precisely what Jim said. The finder of the rifle knew he'd found a treasure with monetary value, and I think he misinterpreted my gesture to indicate possession, or at the very least touching what was his. He would have none of it, and he dissed me thoroughly. Disappointed, I was still intrigued by the rifle and the story.

Mindful of my journalism degree and the pastoral care clergy person I later became, I posed a question to myself: "I wonder what happened to the original owner of that gun? Was he a German invader, or a Russian defender of ancestral soil?"

I still consider these questions. Millions of people died in the German invasion of Russia, the southern thrust of which stormed through this area. Did the soldier who carried the rifle die? Did he live? Which side was he on? Did he return to his family? If not, did his family ever learn what happened to him?

My dear lifetime friend Steve Owen had a keepsake from his father John, a World War II U.S. Army veteran. Mr. O., as I called Steve's dad, was a valiant United States Army tank gunner with the 12th Armored Division who had a bent for history and memorabilia. He removed a belt and buckle from a dead German soldier as a souvenir. The buckle had the words Gott Mittens emblazoned on it. This buckle was a standard issue item to German soldiers. Translated, it means, God be With Us.

Consider the irony of a government regime whose infamy includes the Holocaust of Nazi concentration camps, stamping out such buckles for their Army regulars. Steve knew of my desire to have such a treasure, so he gifted me with the buckle. Why would I want it? Because good German men wore those belt buckles into war. Those Germans were ordinary men turned into soldiers, some of whom were free of being warped by those who ran the

German government and ordered them about. Around their waists they wore a symbol that defied those who tried to indoctrinate them. By keeping their pants, and perhaps their spirits, secure with the buckle, they invoked God for his presence and protection. Shouldn't I do likewise in my life?

My dear friend Steve knew I was a history minor who had an interest in the tiny archives of war. Of the lifetime of countless kindnesses "O" has done for me, giving me this keepsake from his father was so very special. Thanks "O."

On the mountain, I told myself the German soldiers who fought in the Elbrus area would have worn such belts and buckles. I didn't get to hold the gun, but thanks to Steve, I got to wear something special that now meant even more to me by having visited where the German invasion began.

Back at our Barrels base camp about mid-afternoon, after this unusual break in the action, we headed to the kitchen trailer where we took our meals. Leanne, our wonderful cook, did a remarkable job keeping us fed from those blue barrels we lugged up there. We took seats at the table designated for our group and, to my surprise, Jim sat with us. Remarkably, he looked us both in the eye.

"What's up now?" I asked myself. Something had changed. We waited to see what he would do next. Would this turn into an argument or an offer of friendship? Jim began a normal conversation without mention of my snoring or my thoughtless remarks from that morning, when I used the verbal accelerator instead of the brake.

Slowly, his gregarious nature returned and neither of us brought up the earlier incident. We enjoyed dinner and Jim talked engagingly, as before. I thanked God for answering prayers. My bad habit of snoring promoted anger and suffering, which my big mouth exacerbated. I had apologized for both. I said prayers. I also had let it go, having done what I could do. Now, things were as they had been. Thank you, God of mercy.

Later, I told Lori in private, "If I start to snore again, throw a full water bottle across the room immediately, please, right at my head." Thankfully this issue only surfaced for a mili-second and Lori got me to immediately go mute.

During the entire trip I had issues with my Blackberry, from reception failure to dying batteries. The tool meant to be a lifeline home and power a blog to St. Vincent youth obesity donors, was mostly a failure. Arrgh. And much of the trouble rested with the pilot—me. Before the trip my mate Scott Cox at St. Vincent Salem, which had become one of my new ministries, installed some kind of electronic device on the BB.

"With this tool I'll always know where you and Lori are. I'll know your whereabouts within 600 feet at all times—as long as you have the Blackberry on you," he said. Scott was a U.S. Navy veteran with intelligence experience who shared my concerns about issues in Russia that ranged from politics to crevasses. I wanted us to be safe on the slopes and on the streets—Scott helped us with that.

As I went to bed, the Blackberry logged an email from South Bend, IN, from a woman I met at grief training in Colorado. Oh, geez—not now! I switched the BB to off. For all its problems, it seemed to work for that particular message. Crazy.

Thursday, June 24, 2010

Dominic and Kathryn's 10th Anniversary

All three of us—Jim, Lori and I—slept around the clock. Jim stepped from his area in front of our Barrel 7 with a hardy "Morning, Walter!" What a difference from 24 hours earlier. Thanks again, God for answering my prayers.

On the other side of the room Lori continued snoozing. First thing, I wished my older son and his wife a happy anniversary. Other morning activities after Scripture time included drinking a liter of water, catching up my journal, and looking at pictures in my journal of my lovely family: Andy and Jill, and Dom and Kathryn, and their lovely Siena—my granddaughter. And I longed to see them. My morning ritual also included an important visit to the loo. Visits there always reminded me of what we take for granted in the comfort and privacy of our own homes. The loo was smelly, dirty, and contained no toilet paper (we brought our own). The only available hygiene came from the hand sanitizers or moist towlettes we carried ourselves. Waste dropped into a shallow hole. This loo had a kind of seat made of 2x4 wood pieces, but sometimes there isn't a seat and one must improvise for comfort, safety (lest you fall in), and effectiveness (as in aim). Often the next customers impatiently lurk outside the door. This loo was about 200 steps from our quarters, so timing was important to outrace the others. I didn't like to wait. With support staff, about 30 people shared Base Camp and its single seat loo serving both genders. No wonder we often had to wait. One positive note: To the left of this primitive bathroom was a majestic view of the Caucasus Mountains looking east. Usually we saw the sunrise. Alas, not today, as it was snowing. To the west we'd been observing the full moon, but not on this day, given the weather.

Snow had fallen overnight and continued to fall as we went to the trailer for breakfast.

Hot porridge awaited us from LeeAnna, plus fruit, chocolate, and the dark bread. She also proudly provided a dish of golden caviar, a primo specialty version of this Russian seafood delicacy. After trying it, I needed more hot chocolate, instant coffee, and my water with Gatorade powder added. The disagreeable taste lingered, but I was happy I tried the caviar. Having this premium golden caviar available is important to Russians hosting foreigners to their homeland. I like most all food, but this caviar was something my taste buds never got used to. Probably a good thing methinks—it would be an expensive taste to cultivate.

Jim's charming conversational skill continued to shine as we ate breakfast, and I felt quietly grateful we are back to normal. Sergey dismissed us right after the meal, but wanted us to return directly after freshening up. We would be outfitted and prepared for a training session on ice axe arrest during this, our final day of training. Early the next morning we would head for the summit.

The snow continued to fall as we headed to a short, steep slope to learn about using ice axes, something new to Lori and I. Jim already knew the techniques. Sergey instructed us for more than two hours as the snowfall continued. Ice axe use is essential to stop falling on a slope. The trick is, while falling, to drag the pick's sharp end through the snow to slow and stop the fall and avoid injury, or worse.

The proper method for using the ice axe has a climber place it safely underneath his (or her) chest to put body weight atop it to make the pick go into the snow to provide arrest—that is, slow and stop the sliding. We learned how to do this while at the same time getting our bodies in proper position to leverage the axe. You don't want the axe inadvertently impaling an arm, leg, chest cavity, or face. And of course as we would perform this while sliding downhill and maneuvering our bodies to simultaneously position the axe. Not to mention the fear factor and adrenaline surge involved with sliding. If you don't do this correctly in a real life situation you will find yourself in harm's way, from the axe and from the slide. When you're tied into a rope with your fellow climbers a fall becomes more serious because other climbers are at risk. Did I mention this requires coordination, strength, agility, and poise?

Jim was good to go with his axe, having trained before. I gave Lori and myself grades of B or B- on this skill. "Dear God, that we don't need to use these things," I prayed.

Our geographic position was at 43 degrees latitude—40 degrees different from where I climbed at Kilimanjaro just south of the equator. We were less than two miles from the Georgia border and 100 miles from the Black Sea, the lowest point in Russia. I found it interesting that the highest and lowest points in Russia were neighbors, close as a round-trip drive from Columbus to Indianapolis. Mt. Elbrus is the highest point in Russia, and it is said that a on a clear day one could view in one direction the Black Sea, Russia's lowest point, and in the opposite direction, the Caspian Sea.

The Black Sea coastal town of Sochi would host the future Winter Olympics in four years—2014. Soon afterward, the embattled region of Crimea, a day's drive from Sochi, would become a de facto warzone. These areas formed the backyard of the Russian state of Georgia and environs. They were tinderboxes for radical religious insurgents, and also for land grabs by Moscow leaders. This was home to the Caucasus Mountains where we climbed. From the top of Russia's Elbrus we didn't see either the Black or Caspian Sea. But later we would witness the politics and combativeness of the region.

We spend the afternoon packing and re-packing gear for our climb to—God willing—the roof of Russia, the highest point on continental Europe. Except that a "maybe" had surfaced. Make that "Maybe times two."

Maybe 1:

Lori had a crisis of confidence. The way I saw it, she became keenly aware mountain climbing was dangerous. I talked and talked about that during our training, but she minimized my warnings.

Now, she felt uncertain about safely making the climb. Fear seized her mind, causing her to worry about her safety and whether she had the strength to climb the mountain. At home, she had two teen-age daughters who needed her. She was ready to withdraw from the climb.

Speaking candidly, I told her, "I don't want to blow sunshine up your butt, but I'm confident you have the strength to make the summit and back, safely." Nonetheless, I told her it was prudent to be concerned about her safety, and for everyone's safety.

This climb would not be a walk in the park. Mt. Elbrus is challenging. As mountain guides say, about one per cent of the population do what we were about to do. I advised her that if she wanted to sit it out, I'd be okay with that. There's no shame or disgrace in making a decision based on facts. That would be a courageous move, I said. Wanting to empower her, I added, "But if you choose not to climb because you think you aren't strong enough, then your choice is poorly grounded."

More tears, and more indecision.

About this time Jim came into The Barrel. He sensed something was up and asked us, "What's wrong?"

Despite the one rough day, we had jelled as a team. I glanced at Lori. This was her announcement to make, not mine. I wasn't going to violate her privacy. But Lori spoke openly about her fears and tearfully outlined the problem. When she finished speaking, and only then, did I say my piece about believing she had the strength to do this.

Jim was an international airplane pilot—and pilots tend to be take-charge people. They need that personality trait because of what they do. So Jim took charge. He bordered perhaps on being overbearing, but managed not to be. His position clearly and succinctly stated was that: "You should make the climb. I had doubts about your ability when you first got to the mountain, but your performance has taken care of that."

Like me, he encouraged Lori. How would this turn out, I wondered?

Maybe 2.

Sergey came to our Barrel a bit later, looking grim from the bad weather news he was about to deliver in his broken English. He said snow had been coming down all night and all day in our immediate area of the mountain. Not good. Worse, the higher elevations also experienced snowfall. There was no way to sugar coat this, in broken English or perfect English.

"If the snow it continues to fall, we not climb."

And the weather forecast was bleak: The snow was supposed to continue. Sergey said he would monitor the weather alerts between now and 3 a.m., the time scheduled for our wake-up call. At three in the morning he would give us the "Go" or "No Go" when he came to our barrel. He looked at us for questions. The situation was black and white, so we found nothing to ask him. He summarized the news and it would turn out good or bad. Sergey left.

Now it became time for me to take charge.

Looking at Jim, I asked, "Do you mind if I say a prayer? I want to say a prayer for weather and the opportunity to climb."

Jim nodded. "Go ahead."

I looked at Lori, who had heard me pray and speak of praying many, many times. She also nodded.

"Dear God, I pray within your will. I don't want to be selfish, but if the mountain doesn't need this snow right now, will you please bring it to an end? I'd like for us to have a shot at the summit and for that to happen, we need a change in the weather. Thank you, God. Amen."

As I finished, a bright stream of sunshine abruptly pierced through our Barrels' window. This was the first sunlight we'd seen all day. And through that small window we saw the snowflakes had stopped falling.

Honestly, the weather change happened just like that.

Jim smiled and exclaimed, "Keep saying that prayer!"

Quietly, I responded. "I will, and I want you to keep praying also."

Lori reconsidered and said she would make the climb.

Maybe 1 – Lori said it was a "go" for her!

Maybe 2– Prayers were underway. In fact, it wasn't just prayers from Barrel 7. On all my climbs, I ask my prayer warrior friends and program donors to pray for expedition safety, favorable weather, and summit success. So I knew many people were enjoined in this prayer. We would know the results at 3 a.m. when next we saw Sergey: Go or no-go.

Friday, June 25, 2010

Climbing Day, and Dominic's 39th birthday

My son Dom's birthday is today. Happy 39th to you!

But this day, the three of us received the first present (remember Russia is nine hours ahead of Indiana, where it was still yesterday). At 3 a.m. sharp, Sergey knocked on Barrel 7's door and let himself in. I was awake. I called over to Lori and could hear Jim awakening. We quickly gathered to await the news.

"So, well," Sergey began in in his customary way of starting a sentence, "I don't know what happen, but the snow it is stopped. The weather report looks okay. But there is chance of snow. So we go. Get ready now. LeeAnna is make breakfast." Sergey always kept things short, and often sweet.

"Thank you God for hearing the weather payer," said I. I also said, "Hallelujah! Praise the Lord and rock and roll!"

Jim followed, exclaiming, "Showtime!"

Lori "amened" it all, saying "Alright!"

The barrel had little heating, so I was already partially dressed and pulled on enough clothes for the trip to the loo, and then to the trailer for breakfast. Yesterday Sergey had said if the forecasted winds moved to higher elevations, the wind chill would make the air seem like -21 degrees below Fahrenheit up top. I thanked God again because, as at least here, the winds were calm.

We ate without saying much because we are all focusing, and we needed to be ready. A snow cat would move us a few hundred feet higher on the mountain and we wanted to be waiting when it arrived.

Roxanne joined us, a new player to the cast, our auxiliary guide we had just met yesterday. She was summoned as the result of the difference of opinion between Jim and I. Jim felt we'd be adequately protected by having only Sergey. I disagreed, saying if anything happened to Sergey, as healthy as he was, we would be left with a guide to care for, plus ourselves, on a mountain that's 18,513 feet high and the temp might feel like -20 below zero. Plus, if we got into trouble he was one and we were three.

I asked Jim to consider his tolerance for risk with his aircraft, crew, and passengers. What standards did he follow as a pilot? I said: "And, I know it'll cost more money, but that's money well spent."

I appreciated that Jim listened and I felt grateful for his deference to my position. So Roxanne was summoned by Sergey from our outfitter. She was from the mountains, the wine and beef country of Argentina near South America's Seven Summit mountain Mount Aconcagua where I would climb in 18 months. A small, young, wiry woman, she was pleasant. "You can call me Roxie, you know like those rocks," she said pointing to the ground. Her English was good, which I thought was an added bonus.

We finished eating and returned to #7 to complete our preparations. Sergey and Roxie soon arrived at our doorstep.

Now we were five, complete and awaiting the Snow Cat. Lori suddenly discovered her trek poles were missing, having left them in The Barrel which was already padlocked and the big key given to LeeAnna.

"Oh, geez," I muttered. I dashed to the dining trailer and got the key from LeeAnna. Lori got her trek poles, and the Cat pulled up. Unfortunately, Lori unwittingly left behind one of her water bottles. This would cost us on our descent.

The Snow Cat dropped us a few hundred feet up the mountain. The smell of the diesel engine exhaust reminded me of the diesel engine products Cummins Engine manufactures in my community. We were seated as on the bed of a pickup truck like Snow Cat that was noisy, smelly, and cramped. I felt the cold air as we moved along about 20 miles an hour. The ride didn't last long.

We started climbing a little before 4:30 a.m. and would ascend for nine hours. Shouldering our packs, we steadily moved up the mountain. The clouds were gone for now and we had a full luna or moon, surrounded by vivid stars in an inky black sky. Up we went. Lori was moving smoothly, as was Jim, following Sergay.

Something seemed to be pulling at me, and I couldn't figure out what it was. It felt like a constriction. By our first rest stop, with Roxi's help I figured it out. The tightness was restricting my ability to cleanly move my legs to climb. My steps felt bound, like I was hamstrung. I asked Roxi to adjust the straps on my climbing harness which vertically connected the waist belt to the leg loops. At Base Camp when she set them she'd gotten these so tight they were binding me and making my steps much more difficult than necessary. Once loosened, I was free of the constriction and able to move with customary climbing ease. Wow, what a freedom that was. Now the 25 pound back pack load seemed much lighter and I fancied I even had some spring in my step.

The sun came out, praise the Lord. We saw only a wispy cloud to the west over Georgia way. What a harbinger for the future that cloud would become. Steadily up Elbrus we went. Thank you, God for my body, mind and spirit. I felt, as it were, at one with the mountain. We took breaks pretty much on the hour. We were somewhat together as a group, un-roped in this section. Roxie brought up the rear, for some of the day, with Jim now in front of her, then Lori, me, and Sergey in the lead. The pace was comfortable—not racing and not plodding.

Because Sergey held the world record on Elbrus for the fastest ascent and descent, to a sprinter or thoroughbred like him, our collective pace must have resembled one of the Russian cows I saw ambling along the road during the drive to the mountain.

Toward midmorning we made a wide traverse around the mountain to the west. We were moving now from the east mountain to the west mountain, whose higher summit we sought. The transition was significant in a couple of ways. As we gained a saddle or plateau, we took a break. Following restroom relief, hydration, and a snack, we put on our crampons.

We eliminated into a ground cache and temporarily left everything behind we didn't need in our packs for the final push, like extra water and food meant for our descent. We traded trek poles for ice axes, shouldered the lighter packs, and resumed what was now a steep climb. I guessed at this point we were perhaps three, maybe two, hours from the summit. As we gained elevation, mountain tops appeared below us.

And as we looked up, the transition that began on the plateau further unfolded. The wisp of cloud to the west now became a cloud deck we were climbing toward. Up and up we went, the terrain becoming more challenging as it grew steeper. I asked Lori how she was going along. Lori said she was okay. I kept trying to match my steps to Sergey's ahead of me, kicking my steps where his feet had been. The crampons enabled us to kick a good stepping platform in the snow. I noticed Jim had fallen behind. I didn't know if he slowed intentionally or not. Roxie was behind him. As we continued to ascend, it seemed he'd gotten farther back. I didn't expect he was weakening, but who knows? All I knew was that he lagged further behind us. I mentioned this to Sergey and his answer was, "Roxie is with him."

We stood high above Russia at some 17,000 feet, near a steep outcropping that offered a break from climbing. Remembering Sergey's speed record, I teased him about how slowly he had to move with us. In response, a tiny smile creased his lips.

I followed him onto the rocks and found one I could straddle, with my butt up the mountain from the rocky mass and my legs astride it. The steepness of the mountain was such that I could securely wedge my cramponed boot heels into the snow-covered icy glacier. Fairly comfortable, I felt secure with this seating arrangement. A minute later when my climbing partner Lori pulled in and I helped her get safely squared away. I added slowly and carefully, "If you take off your pack, anchor it above and behind that rock." A loose pack would slide all the way back to the plateau where we'd stowed gear a thousand sharply angled feet below.

An amazing panorama lay before us. Russia's Caucasus range stretched in all directions and we were higher than all the snow covered peaks in sight. We were also above the cloud deck, but the clouds were moving, our sunlight becoming eclipsed. I told myself this scene might have been around since the Creation days, after the continental shifts, after these volcanoes bowed out to their curtain-call explosions. What a majestic timeless vista Elohim the

Creator God gave us to behold. I said some of this to Lori, telling her to treasure the view in her heart. What she said in response still makes me laugh out loud.

Lori quietly took in the incredible view, then turned back to me and said, "You know I'm scared of heights don't you?"

Incredulous, I almost blurted, "You're joking!" When I realized she was serious, my eyes nearly bugged out of my head.

"Yeah, at home I won't even climb on a ladder to paint the garage or clean the gutters,"

Realizing she meant every word, I thought better of laughing. I was torn between telling her, "Don't look down," or saying, "Maybe those clouds will move in to hide the view." Instead, I managed to mutter: "Well, enjoy lunch." An hour later I would regret wishing for clouds.

Later, when I asked Lori about this she spoke of the mom of a cerebral palsy patient she cared for—how the mother and her son faced their fears. This wise woman taught herself, her son, and Lori it was okay to be frightened, but then we need to face our fears. The mom had a rock inscribed with *No Fear*. That thinking empowered Lori at sea level, but today at 17,000 feet she went breathless as she gazed at the world below us. She said she didn't consciously hide her fear from me—she felt she could handle it by herself, and she did, until that moment of sharing.

Above us loomed 1,000 vertical feet to the Roof of Russia. At 18,513 feet (3.5 miles high), Mount Elbrus towers above the surrounding terrain. High winds, cold nights, a long summit day, and unpredictable weather make Elbrus a difficult climb with a high failure rate. But things were looking good for us, with only 90 minutes of climbing to reach the summit.

Awaiting our companions James and Roxanne, we munched apples, ate chocolate and cheese, and hydrated. The water tasted good—later I would remember how good. We'd been going up since before 4 a.m. after awakening at 3 a.m. Soon it would be noon. I enjoyed having the pack off. Even though we'd jettisoned gear down below and the pack was lighter, any weight felt heavy eight hours later, at this altitude.

Our companions arrived 15 minutes later, maybe longer. Nothing was said about their pace. The mountain's "aspect," how mountaineers refer to a slope's angle, was steep on the last 1,000 feet. That steepness would continue, and it slowed Jim's pace.

When everyone finished eating we prepared for the final push up to the summit.

Sergey pulled a tan rope coil from his backpack and stretched it out. Time for us to rope up. We each tied the rope into the harnesses we wore around our waists—and then attached that rope to the climber ahead of us and behind us. The mountaineering trope is: The Brotherhood of the Rope. Sergey led, then Jim, me, Lori, and Roxie. We were now a rope team. As such our cadence, or dance steps as I called it, needed to be in alignment and timed so we were all walking in synch.

Upward we went, climbing steadily while trying for roped rhythm. A wrong step would cause the ropes to go too taut or too slack. Either way, an out-of-step climber threw off one or more of his partners. I'd spent much of the last eight hours walking behind Sergey and I had his pace dialed in. Jim moved a tick slower. For a while I found myself going a wee bit faster and bumped into him. Not that I needed this brought to my attention, but Jim brought it to my attention. Sometimes with a growl. I didn't blame him. In addition to my bumps annoying him, we were all fatigued after climbing for several hours. Jim didn't need his physical and emotional equilibrium thrown off by the guy behind him. After a few more bumps and complaints, thankfully, I adapted to his pace.

Consider our burdens: We each wore layered clothing for warmth and carried a weighted backpack. We wore 12-point crampons tied to each foot over our big heavy boots. For additional safety we carried the ice axes to arrest a fall. Ski goggles covered our faces.

And soon we were walking into a whiteout as the cloud deck began to envelop us. Then snow began to fall. Tiny flakes like powdered sugar danced in the air. Beautiful, but not exactly a walk in the park.

Bump!

"Walter—watch it!" Jim growled.

"Sorry, Jim."

When the clouds totally engulfed us and the landscape became veiled, I regretted my earlier thoughts about clouds moving in. Now, the clouds merged so perfectly with the mountain that I could scarcely see where to place my feet. The snow increased as we steadily ascended. Our crampons and ice axes bit into the glacier's hard surface. Thankfully, no one slipped or fell. We each moved efficiently. There was something of a trail from other climbers, although here on the upper mountain not another soul was in sight. Not one. Come to think of it, the last guy we'd seen hours ago was headed down—right after sunrise. He must have overnighted in a bivouac on the mountain.

The higher we went, the more socked in the terrain became, with the cloud cover and falling snow increasing. But we were nearing our goal, our quest during those long months of training. I felt a surge of joy when Sergey told Jim, who passed the word to me and on down the line, "We're getting close, about 15 minutes from the summit."

The worsening conditions made it nearly impossible to see. Visibility ahead was down to 20 feet. We couldn't see the summit, and in fact the white of the mountain's surface blended into the cloudy surroundings, producing a few missteps.

Sergey paused our rope team at a compacted, level clearing. Jim closed in on Sergey, as did I, and then the women. Sergey stretched out his carbide-tipped trek pole and slowly waved it over his head. The theologian in me imagined Moses waving his staff. I started to tease Sergey, asking if he were going to part the clouds like Moses did the sea. Sergey was not amused.

Not in the mood for a Biblical reference, Segey continued holding up his trek pole, the metallic end pointing skyward, and the handgrip near his face. He looked at me with a steely gaze and commanded, "Walter, Listen."

He thrust the trek pole handle near my ear. I heard buzzing and crackling. Like Ben Franklin of legend with a key on a kite string, Sergey was monitoring weather in the air, specifically electricity. The metal end of his trek pole attracted the electricity and produced the static sound.

For reference, consider the legend of Ben Franklin putting a kite aloft into a colonial era thunderstorm. As the story goes, the kite string had a skeleton key tied to it and that key attracted lightening.

In the few seconds I had to process this, our climb came to a screeching and non-negotiable halt. Sergey said: "We are in electric storm. I am sorry. I send you down with Roxanne for safety."

What the guide says on a mountain is law. We signed an agreement saying so. Like that, our Elbrus adventure came to a close. Yet, as Lori and I turned to leave, Sergey and James continued up the mountain without us. What was up with those two, I asked myself, feeling angry and frustrated. I honestly didn't know why it was okay for them to continue upward; I never asked.

I did know an electrical storm was serious at the top of the world. I knew I had children and a grandchild. Lori had daughters. We valued our lives, and our families expected us to come back alive. Neither of us needed to be within range of a zap-and-fry electrical storm. Sergey and James were adults, single men. They could do what they wanted.

Why was I furious? Well, who do you think is in charge of weather? I was mad at God! Why? Because we trained our butts off to be here. Because we climbed all day to be within minutes of the summit. We were raising money for a noble cause—diminishing childhood obesity. Plus, Lori and I each paid a pretty penny from our own pockets to be in Russia.

And now we were thwarted by weather, with the prize almost in reach. No summit? I was steamed at God, the ultimate weatherman!

We needed a miracle.

Stunned, I realized we were a mere 15 minutes from the prize, only to hear the climb was over. Even worse, we were now in a danger zone. The chance of snow Segrey mentioned in his weather report at three a.m. had become a genuine dumping, with clouds creating a near total white-out. But those occupational hazards on a mountain climb were to be expected, accepted, and overcome.

The electrical storm was not a typical hazard, and because of it, we were being ordered down the mountain. Yet, Jim would continue upward. Did he cut a private deal with Sergey? I never asked. We needed to turn around, go downward with Roxie, and be safe. Let me be clear: I wasn't envious of Jim. Perhaps Sergey thought Jim's climbing experience made him stronger and swifter than Lori and I. Perhaps Jim offered a cash bonus. None of that mattered to me. I am a risk taker by nature, but I didn't fancy being electrocuted.

In spite of all that, I was still fuming. Lori and I trained diligently for this mountain, working hard to be in the best shape to climb this Russian bear. I had trained daily—not missing a single day— since before Christmas. Lori's training schedule meant she only missed a few days. Now we were being kicked down the mountain without an opportunity to prove our mettle. I was pissed. I was pissed at God, the weather, and the circumstances. Lori and I each spent $5,000 of our own money to be there. Our purpose went beyond the adventure; we were raising money and awareness for St. Vincent Jennings to fund the youth obesity L.I.F.E for Kids prevention and treatment program, and for her Peyton Manning Children's Hospital at St. Vincent. I was, excuse my French, Pissed with a capital P.

Two of my mentors, Father Adrian VanKaam and Susan Muto of the Epiphany Center in Pittsburgh, speak of our two natures: the Christ-form, and the pride-form. At that point, my pride held sway—I admit that. But darn, we were trying to do good with our efforts on the mountain. Dozens of people had asked for blessings on our behalf, including weather prayers, and many others took the next step and financially supported this climb.

"And here, God, you let this storm blow in. And we are stopped." Of course, Elbrus is known to harbor some of the most unpredictable weather on the planet. Unusual is the norm. My passion was over-ruling my spirituality and faith. And I realized it.

Time to grow up; time to put the brakes on my reckless ranting and emotional whining. Weather had precluded our summit attempt. We were thwarted, not by inability, but by something greater than ourselves. A mature spiritual person can complain, I reasoned. And I certainly did so. However, to enflesh the blame and direct it at God, to give it formation as an attitude and let the emotion rule me would to ruin this entire experience. I had bitched and whined for a short time. Okay. Done.

"Now, I really need to let go of this," I told myself, "My prayer in Barrel 7 was introduced by "Praying within God's will.""

I continued the lecture: "Walter, you need to let it go. The inclement weather must be God's will. So, please grow up and be a mature spiritual person. Let it go. Enough, already. Done. God, forgive me—please. More later. Right now I need to focus."

And I did let it go. No matter the summit, I thought back to my morning prayer: "I will greet the new sun with confidence that this will be the best day of my life." Somewhere the sun was shining. It was time to let the sun re-shine in my heart. We would celebrate all the good of this expedition, and already there was plenty of good.

As I let go and stopped fuming, I felt the tension, angst, and darkness leave my heart. I felt good, or at least better. Now, having pitched a fit, and moreover healing it, I felt ready to down climb. I had my temper tantrum. So be it. Jesus did the same in his Father's house when he turned the business world of the temple upside down, literally, with his temple temper tantrum. He was angry, but he didn't let the anger rule him. Nor would I. Mustering all the suppleness and docility that lay within me, I let go of the anger and angst constricting me, just as the climbing harness strap had earlier been loosened. I loosened the bonds that tied me up. I was free of it and felt lighter.

Then I heard a familiar sound from a few days earlier during our training—a sharp, piercing whistle from Sergey. Lori, Roxie, and I stopped in our tracks and turned 180 degrees to look up mountain. And there, in a remarkable clearing among the vaporous clouds and snowfall, stood Sergey and James. Somehow the shroud-like snowfall and clouds parted enough for us to see Sergey waving us to return.

Hardly believing this wonderful blessing, I turned and plodded upward again. When we reached Sergey and gave him questioning looks, he didn't say much. True to his nature, he was brief in his broken English. "I know not what happen, but the storm it has passed. The electric is gone. We go up now. And we hurry. Maybe storm return, maybe no. But it is snowing. Snow falling hard. Only a few minutes now from top. We hurry—danger on way down. Only be a few minutes there, and back down. Hurry now."

With Sergey's brief instruction, just like that, we returned to the ascent. The green flag of racing, as it were, had dropped.

"What happened to the electrical storm?" people often ask me.

"I don't know" I say.

"Do you believe your change of heart changed the weather?"

"I don't know," I say.

"Do you think that weather change was just a meteorological coincidence?"

"Well, I don't really believe in coincidences," I say.

"Well, then, what happened?"

And the routine goes on. I cannot answer those questions; I can only report and summarize what happened:

a) Just below about 18,500 feet of elevation on Mount Elbrus in Russia we climbed into an electrical storm on crampons fabricated from metal and held carbide tipped trek poles in our hands—we could easily become human lightning rods;

b) A thick cloud deck and snowstorm mere minutes and meters from the summit produced near whiteout conditions;

c) My two responses to the weather were: Anger, pride, pouting, possibly a bit of self-righteous indignation; and then, ultimately—some maturity. Was there a correlation between the change in the weather and the change in my heart? I cannot answer that conclusively.

d) What I do know is this: After the interior change in me, our outside environment changed. What I do know is, I had prayed in God's will and prayed about the weather, safety, and summit success. Many other people were praying for the same things, on our behalf. I believe prayer changes people, and people change things. Can people change the weather? I believe a meteorologist would say, "Of course not."

So, was this a miracle? I think not. Miracles happen when circumstances change without a plausible, scientific reason. I do know that a wonderful change in the weather coincided with a wonderful change that occurred in me.

As we climbed, the snow turned to huge flakes that resembled powdered sugar being shaken from a bag. A line in Psalms describes how "God sews the snow as wool." Wool, powdered sugar— whatever God was sewing, and the snowfall came dense and fast.

We still couldn't see the summit, but Sergey announced we were five minutes away. I began crying, sobbing out loud in fact—and these were tears of joy. In crampons, carrying an ice axe, wearing a 25 pound back pack, I suddenly began to out-distance my superbly fit partner.

Lori called to me to, "Hey, slow down! You know, 'poley poley.'" Talk about a role reversal.

During the last minutes, I made the climb on my hands and knees, using the ice axe for purchase on the final steep and slick section. I was close enough now to see Jim, Roxie, and Sergey up top. I waited for Lori just short of the crest and we summited together. Then we grabbed Jim and Sergey with whoops and hollering LeeAnna might have heard down at The Barrels. We exchanged high fives and hugs, collectively and in pairs—even Sergey, the reticent Russian. I said a prayer of thanksgiving. Next, time for the celebratory photo shoot. I unfurled a banner for St. Vincent Jennings and Lori pulled out a T-shirt with the name of Peyton Manning Children's Hospital at St. Vincent. We later joked that Peyton Manning the Colts' quarterback, despite his superb athletic accomplishments, had never been so high up. The puffy, popcorn-sized powdered sugar snowflakes appear in our summit picture on the book cover.

Sergey reigned in the celebration, which lasted only three to four minutes. "So, well. Let us go. The weather, you know."

And with that, our down climb began. Nothing was or would be easy in Russia. This proved true of the descent. As we started again, my euphoria was tempered when I realized how tired my body felt. My knees were knackered and my whole body seemed spent. But as my mountaineering hero Ed Viesturs says, "Getting up is optional. Getting down safely is mandatory."

We started our climb about 4 a.m. and it took us nine hours to summit, arriving at 1:25 p.m. We would require another five hours to return to The Barrels. Especially in the beginning, the descent was very tedious. The falling snow required Sergey, as the lead climber of a rope team, to set belays. He would establish an anchor point with his ice axe by poking and planting it firmly until it held fast in the glacier snow and ice. Then, he tied one end of the rope onto his ice axe and connected us to each other by the rope. We'd use our ice axes and climb down until all the slack of the rope played out. At that point, while the rest the team stood in place, Sergey would pull his axe and down climb to us.

He would set up another anchor point and we repeated the process. We spent about an hour moving down the technical section of Elbrus in this manner, back toward where we had lunch. This was a slow process, but a safe one. I absolutely hurt all over. Lori, on the other hand, continued to move fairly well, as she had all day. Jim too was going along pretty well. Putting one boot in front of the other consumed me. I also needed to concentrate on my breathing. I was glad for Roxie's presence as a guide to help lead the belays. I had never been on a belay, nor had Lori. If we faltered, Roxie was there to coach us.

Down we continued to where we cached our gear in the saddle area. We stowed crampons and ice axes in the packs and returned to using our trek poles. We hydrated. I finished a fourth liter of water. We had, as I remembered, another two hours and more ahead of us. Lori and I didn't know just yet that one precious full bottle of refreshing water was left at Barrel 7.

Away from the higher elevations, the snowfall eased and then stopped. Down, down, down, we went. The cloud deck slowly evaporated, though gray clouds remained overhead. My balance felt a little off as the result of my fatigue. I kept plodding on, with no crispness to my step. Again, Lori moved fine, her fitness and strength shining through. I thought I could see the point where the snowcat vehicle had dropped us in the pre-dawn early morning, but I was mistaken. Alas, it would be awhile before we reached there.

The glacier was pretty much void of topography. What I tried to do was find a point, say a rock or snow mound, and down climb to it. Then I'd find another point and descend to that. This practice helped section the monotony of down climbing for me. I felt a semblance of achievement every few minutes as I reached another mini-goal.

Gradually, the day seemed brighter. That seemed weird to my eyes, as all we'd seen for several hours was gray sky, mountain white, the enveloping clouds and snow, and then more gray. I realized sunlight had begun easing through the gray clouds. The whiteout had lifted. What a perfect time for this gift! The sunlight lifted my spirits. What a weather day we had: Sun, clouds, snow, a whiteout, an electrical storm, big fluffy snow, and now the sun re-emerging to brighten the landscape.

As I walked, I noticed some of my steps set off tiny snow slides that would roll softball-size, picking up a little extra snow here and there before the gravity pull played out. Sunlight beaming on the fresh, wet snowfall sparkled like a million diamonds. Suddenly, the clouds pulled back to reveal the Caucasus Mountains as a backdrop. The mini-avalanches from my boot steps, the sparkling snow diamonds, the mountains' rugged beauty—I spoke to Lori about all of this as we went down, down, down.

"Take this in, don't miss it," I said with some inflection in my voice instead of the tired monotone I heard crawl out of my mouth for the last hour.

Lori told me later she thought maybe I was hallucinating, or at the very least, losing focus.

"Count your steps," she'd say. "How many steps did you get in that last minute?"

All I could do was laugh weakly. I didn't want her to miss God's beautiful creation. Her concern for my welfare led her to mention step-counting.

Throughout the down climb, Lori kept encouraging me. Don't we all appreciate someone to care for us, express concern, and offer encouragement? And I needed such affirmation on the descent. Knowing someone cares about us, especially when the going gets arduous, is a good feeling. And positive energy motivates. This was all helpful to me.

At one stop during a break, I recall Roxie working with me on meditation and breath. Little did she know of my interest in this subject, having often practiced meditation and focus breathing. Again, a helping hand was extended to make my journey easier.

We drained our last sips of water. For me that meant I drank four liters of water, the most ever on a summit day. I could have consumed another liter. In a little while I asked Lori to share her last bottle with me. That's when we discovered she'd left a liter of water in Barrel 7. Part of me wanted to be upset, but I was almost too tired for that. And what would it gain to get mad? She made an honest mistake. Besides, as climbing leader, I should've had a mental checklist to review with my protégé about her preparations, including having X number of liters of water in our packs—and noticing and asking about her missing trek poles. But that was then and this was now. My voice was getting a little raspy from thirst, and Lori also was thirsty.

I used to take care of thirst when I was skiing by eating snow—until I got a case of giardia. Clean-looking snow can collect this parasite from birds or their crap. I understand rain can transmit something akin to this. Diarrhea, intestinal discomfort, and cramps result from giardia. I knew this well, after having all these symptoms during a ski trip at Aspen and thinking I might have appendicitis. After that, I stopped eating snow—and especially not in Russia when we were on a mountain, far from medical relief. So we slogged on without water for what seemed a long time. I expect I grumbled, but honestly I don't remember.

All of us, except Sergey I believe, finished our last drops of water 60 to 90 minutes before taking our final steps on the mountain. This made for an unpleasant final hour. The sun, which seemed so welcome at first, made us warmer and more parched. I'd never drunk more than three liters of water on a summit day, so I wasn't unprepared. But 14 hours made for a long climb. The other time I was out this long on a mountain, Kilimanjaro, our down climb took us back through our camp, where we stopped to refill our water bottles.

Toward the end of Elbrus (would it ever end?) I fell a couple of times. When I needed a hand getting up, Lori was there, or Roxie. Sergey brought up the rear, and Jim now walked in front. More plodding downward, more thirst. I was totally spent, having exhausted my last ounces of energy. I ran on fumes and could hardly talk. I mused that some people would appreciate me being quiet, and the thought made me laugh—but not out loud.

Then, in the distance, down mountain in a flat area I spotted the snow cat waiting to collect us and ferry us across the last section back to The Barrels. Sergey had called the operators on a cell phone to alert them before our arrival. We were another 20 minutes away, I figured. Our ordeal was coming to a close and soon my body could rest and I would quench my thirst. Soon the heavy backpack and the boots would come off, along with all those sweaty clothes. Not having enough water had risen to a real concern, making me ponder yet another thing we take for granted—the immediate availability of clean, pure water from a tap, sometimes made cold with ice cubes.

As we reached, the cat, Lori and I tiredly gave each other, and James, a congratulatory hug—also Sergay and Roxie. We boarded the cat. Lori almost put her hand on the vertical exhaust stack before the driver yelled her away, she having thought it a support handle. Climbing up onto the cat were the final up steps I would make that day—thankfully. The rest and ride back were so helpful to my knackered legs. In a few minutes we returned to Barrel 7, exhausted yet joyful. For me and for James, another one of the Seven Summits was in the bag. And I was delighted for Lori. Sergey must have yearned for his speed record days after enduring all of us!

When we climbed down from the cat our wonderful cook LeeAnna ran right up to me, gave me a big but gentle hug, and bestowed the traditional Russian kiss on both my cheeks. She was so glad to see me, fussing over me. I realized she liked me. Russians hold so much in, silly me—I had no clue. Maybe she was worried about me, the old one! Her traditional Russian kiss was a memorable touch; never before or since!

I slowly and painfully walked into Barrel 7.

Lori went to the dining trailer to get me tea, and I drank two huge cups. I drank more water with Gatorade mix. As I started shedding clothes the indoor clothes line in our part of the barrel started filling up with my seven upper layers and four lower layers of clothing. Slowly, methodically I shed my sweat-soaked summit clothes and got into dry ones. The sun was setting outside The Barrels' window as I did this. Lori followed suit. I may have made an error, but I passed on dinner. Lori brought me a little something and I ate whatever it was. I thought about journaling—dismissed that. I was utterly spent, exhausted, depleted. Bony-weary, every muscle ached. The other times I felt this wasted, I thought, were after Everest, and after Kilimanjaro. The mountains let you climb them, the Tibetan Buddhist Sherpas say. And the appropriate attitude for doing the climbing is humility and gratitude, as though you were climbing into your mother's lap, they say. I felt humble and grateful. And I ached all over.

In my journal I wrote: "This climb was dedicated to the children and their families of the youth obesity programs at St. Vincent Jennings and Peyton Manning Children's Hospital at St. Vincent, and the competent and compassionate clinicians like Lori who care for them. Thanks God for my body, mind and spirit. I'll have more to write tomorrow. But right now I want to shut my eyes."

And one sentence more for the journal: "P.S. Happy Birthday Dom. This summit's for you, bud. On your day."

And I soon was sound asleep.

Saturday, June 26, 2010

I slept for nine hours and doubt I even moved from 8 p.m. to 5 a.m. I awakened at five to a beautiful full moon shining through the barrel's window. "Hope I didn't snore—doubt Lori would have heard me," I whispered and smiled. Then, more seriously, "Hopefully not Jim, if I did snore." Lori was buried under covers on the other side of the room, and no sound of movement from Jim's area. I stayed quiet while going to the loo. En route, I was treated to a most majestic sunrise and a stunning view of the Caucasus Mountain range. The stark gray and black mountains were tipped with triangles of white snow frosting and glistened in the sun, set against a vivid bluebird sky. A hallelujah moment. I whispered, "Creator God Elohim Maker is your name—thank you for all this. To be standing on a mountain on planet Earth and having touched one of the planet's highest points, and now in front of me your sun, the greater light, before me, and your full moon, the lesser light setting behind me. Amen, and thank you."

Later, we ate LeeAnna's last meal, and off the mountain we'd be going in the next hour. Back at The Barrels I suggested to Lori we "go shopping." Curiously, she looked at me. I handed her one of two grocery plastic bags and we walked about 100 steps from our petroleum tank lodging. There, I began to collect small rocks from Elbrus. Lori quickly got the picture and began to gather her own samples. These rocks from mountains make the best of gifts for family, friends, and people special to each climb. Lori knew me well enough to know I disdained actual shopping, so she got a kick out of this trip to "the mountain's mall."

There would be no down climbing that day. We boarded another of the single rickety chair ski lifts, having had to again await its operator. This served as a bookend ride to our arrival on Mount Elbrus—nice symmetry, minus the armed soldiers. Instead, we saw skiers on lift chairs heading toward us on their way up the mountain—a fun day ahead of them. Two more lifts and down we cruised, including a high speed Poma gondola.

And like that we are off the mountain in mere minutes. What a contrast to yesterday's 15 hours up and down, nine of those hours toiling upward.

Our next stop was the outfitters, where we'd turn in our gear and settle up. Tips were paid then, and I visited my billfold for the first time in days. Payments to the outfitter and the tips represented a more significant withdrawal of rubles than I budgeted. Hiring Roxie as the auxiliary guide added to our expense, but was worth every ruble. After paying other expenses, my reserves were lean. I reminded myself most everything from there to Indiana was prepaid, so we should be able to sneak by. How naïve that would soon sound!

We headed back to our hotel—and, oh, the luxury of it: Furniture, warmth, a carpet on the floor. A room, not a barrel. And plumbing! That meant a real shower! The only dirt and grime I wasn't carrying was the Bartholomew county dirt I brought to the glacier on my crampons. My weary muscles and bones craved gallons of hot water.

Having a connection and cell phone power from the room's electricity, I posted on the blog while Lori napped away the afternoon.

She awakened with unexpected angst and wanted to talk. "Should I have been here?" She asked. I supposed it was a valid question, but after having successfully climbed the mountain in a safe manner, she surprised me.

I told her the answer lay with her on-mountain performance.

However, now that we were down, Lori seemed to have residual, yet real, fear from what she'd been through. I told her that seemed reasonable, but should be considered in light of safely reaching the summit. I acknowledged that Jim expressed concerns about her in the beginning, but after watching her train and realizing her strength, he openly endorsed her during her crisis of confidence meltdown. I added that my response to her post-summit angst was based on observable data:

a) Information from the travel company representing the outfitters (distributed in advance to me) listed criteria that suggested Lori was competent and belonged here. The problem with this was that Jim had info I was not given which suggested more stringent criteria. I knew nothing about Jim's additional information until he shared it—and I shared it with Lori so she'd know what I knew;

b) Lori's training performance on Elbrus led to endorsements from me, Jim, and from Sergey—who would not have allowed her to climb if he had doubts.

c) Her performance on the mountain during the summit was the concluding evidence.

Using Sergey's manner of speaking, I asked Lori: "So, well, why are you Monday morning quarterbacking yourself now, after it was successfully done? I don't understand?" I said honestly. What else could I say? So I shut up. Lori stayed quiet. Had she let it go, I wondered, or would she say more?

The telephone rang, our only phone call to the room, and Sergey announced, "Walter, this is Sergey. Walter, we are waiting on you!"

Some comic relief to give Lori and I a timeout.

Sergey and Jim waited downstairs for our celebratory dinner. Sergey used his personal car for transport to a nice restaurant. My earlier calculations showed we were so low on funds that I needed to forego this. I brought nice clothing as gifts to our guides, in addition to the monetary tips. Originally, I planned to give the clothing with tips at our dinner, but it needed to happen right away, as we would excuse ourselves from dinner.

We had words over this. Lori wanted to celebrate, and so did I. She believed we could spend down what few rubles we had and be all right. I disagreed. I told her, "We have to get to Mineral Vody and on to Moscow and to the USA. We can't do this dinner. We have too few rubles and too few USD. Call me a penny-pincher, but that's how it is."

And maybe to herself she did.

We went downstairs to give our gifts. The refusal became more difficult as Sergey offered to buy our meals. Geez! Sergey, who expressed little emotion during the whole expedition, stepped out like this. It was akin to the traditional Russian kiss on both cheeks our great chef LeeAnna gave me—totally unexpected.

Declining Sergey's offer was difficult, but it helped to understand some mountain economics. The wage native guides earn is perhaps (perhaps not) commiserate with what they do. But that's only a portion of how they earn their living. Tips are what move them up the economic ladder. I didn't want Sergey using my/our tip to buy Lori and I dinner. Was I too analytical? Did my refusal rebuff him? I hope not. I was trying to have some integrity in my decision-making process around our finances, and to protect his income. So I declined his offer to treat us. However, I wanted to thank him by presenting our gifts.

Lori gave him currency and one of her brand new Nalgeen water bottles he'd been eyeing. Likewise, I give currency plus a water bottle, hand-warmers, and a carabiner and rope. Then for him, and for LeeAnna and Roxie, I gave nice golfing and T-shirts from St. Vincent Jennings Hospital. Sergey was grateful. Jim even said, "Nice shirts." As this was my third mountain, I'd learned to plan in advance to recognize the mountain guides with, as it were, "local gifts from my hospitals" in addition to cash. Then I had a surprise gift for Sergey. I had brought along adult diapers in case I might need them on the mountain. This is a subject of almost "too much information." Suffice it to say, they weren't needed. But given my diarrhea situation during our training I gave one of these to Sergey saying, "If you ever have another 62 year old with you on the mountain, this might come in handy." And we all had a big laugh.

Then, God love Jim, with kindness, he complicated dinner decision-making by offering to buy our dinners! Now what should we do? Rightly or wrongly, I declined. Maybe I was tired. And when I say that, I mean me. Lori had excused herself as we made small talk after the gifts presentation. I got up to the room and told Lori of Jim's offer and my response. She reluctantly accepted my decision.

So we ate in the hotel dining room where dinner was part of our pre-paid program. Dinner there received a definitive grade of "F" from both of us. Normally the hotel meals ranged from average to good. The breakfast from which I apparently got diarrhea was another matter entirely. The young, pretty waitress with the nice smile wasn't on duty and her absence made a lackluster meal even worse still. Plus, Lori had found among her things a nice shirt to give her. Bummer.

After picking at our food (which included fish heads–ugh) and trying to gain some caloric value, we went for a walk around the hotel premises. It turned out they had an indoor pool we'd not seen, and we stepped inside to view it. The pool is beautiful, water un-rippled, with no one there for whatever reason. Seemed odd. An older guy was on duty.

And, surprise, there was our charming favorite waitress pulling pool duty as a second job. Lori hand gestured to the woman, who spoke no English, to stay put while she ran to retrieve the shirt. When Lori returned and presented the shirt, the young woman's smile went from pretty to amazingly high beam. She hugged Lori again and again. I stood back, not wanting to commit a cultural faux pas by hugging her—I didn't know the rules of Russia around this.

And so we concluded our first day in six months without training. For me this was six months on the nose, as we began training the day after Christmas, Well, I didn't train on the travel days to Russia and Lori missed a few days. It felt weird not wearing the backpack after my relentless vigilance of daily training. Our training, though, paid off for both of us. Thank you God for our bodies, minds, and spirits, and to be injury-free.

Sunday, June 27, 2010

We had breakfast with gregarious Jim, our last meal together as he would catch the early car to Mineral Vody. He wanted to board the first flight out. The wisdom of a comment he made around the first flight out was lost on me at the time. And we saw him off—a pleasant ending to what could have been a rocky relationship. Jim was thoughtful and weeks later the youth obesity prevention and treatment clinical program at St. Vincent Jennings received a generous donation from him. Thanks, Jim!

Lori and I planned to catch the last flight out from Mineral Vody to Moscow, so we wouldn't leave until afternoon. My thinking: I'd rather spend my last hours in the quiet of the mountain village than arrive early in Moscow and flounder around the huge international airport.

I hoped to step into a mountain village church, as it was Sunday. Perhaps I could even find an Eastern Orthodox Catholic church, which I knew existed in Russia. Alas, according to the hotel staff, our village did not have a single church. The Russian government had exterminated religion and churches in the area, although I understand a sanctioned revival was slowly underway.

As we left the dining room I meet Wally II, the first one having been at the front end our trip when I saw the banner with "Welcome Wally Gomez" on it. This Wally was named Wally Berg, whom I didn't know but recognized immediately as someone I'd seen before.

Have you ever had that happen? You're somewhere far from home and unexpectedly run across someone you recognize, from home or somewhere else. I introduced myself as "Walter" and he answered, "I'm one too, but just Wally."

"I've seen you before," I said, "but I am not sure where. Maybe Colorado in the winter?"

A few questions and answers later, Wally and I determined we were skiing at Copper Mountain, Colorado about the same time and we both frequented a restaurant there called Farley's at the bottom of B Lift.

I told him I remembered the chef's name, Jim Issacson and he was from Indianapolis originally. Wally remembered him too. We had a nice conversation and exchanged business cards. Hours later, Wally would be supportive to Lori and I amid Elbrus Crisis II. Meanwhile, I thought I knew his name another way. His card said he was Wally Berg the "Founding Director" of Berg Adventures International, headquartered in Canmore, Alberta, Canada. His name rang a bell. I later figured it out at home. I dug out a special edition of National Geographic magazine on Mount Everest. Within that issue was a fold-out picture of Everest taken from high on the mountain. The fold-out pic page carried the notation, "Photograph by Wally Berg." The same guy! Cool beans. I still have your card, Wally!

This was supposed be our last morning at the mountain, and we still had a few hours before our shuttle ride to the airport. It was raining when we told Jim farewell, and the rain made a pleasant melody on the metallic roof. About the only other "rainfall" sound I'd heard was in the shower.

After the rain, we had time for a walk, minus backpacks. We walked along the roadbed, and then beside a creek bed. Snowmelt from Elbrus and the surrounding mountains had turned a creek into a rushing river swollen from snow melt. I think of my son Andy, Columbus North High School's Varsity soccer coach, when I see a fairly well maintained soccer field. Here, we walked past a field with rusty antiquated lights mounted on old fashioned standards and nestled against the mountainside. I wondered what Andy would think of playing there. The thought made me feel melancholy, missing Andy and his Jill. I reminisced about the many soccer games I watched him play and coach. What a great kid. Such a great husband. What a great wife. What a fantastic coach. Then I thought of Dom, Kathryn, and Siena, and how remarkable they also were, individually and as a family. And more melancholy moved in. The rain had stopped earlier, but now my eyes grew misty.

My eyes lost their mist and sharpened as I noticed a nice late model car, clean and shiny drive by. The driver glared at us. Minutes later the car returned going the other way and we got the look again from man behind the wheel. Oh, geez, time for the walk to end. We hurried back to the hotel. Lori found me a worrywart at times, but my alert meter from Red Square had suddenly kicked into high gear. Fortunately we didn't see the car again, but we were about to see a lot that didn't look right.

Later, packed and sitting with our luggage in the hotel lobby, we confidently awaited the four hour ride to the Mineral Vody airport. I had tried to buy Russian beer to take home, but alas, night before was Saturday and the locals had a party. The beer refrigerator was empty. I mean out—completely. I inquired of staff to buy beer and I was told, the obvious, "The frig is empty."

"Yes, I can see that. When will you restock it?" I asked.

"Who knows?" was the thickly accented reply. Having learned Russian body language for "frustration," I threw up my hands and frowned. So did the woman behind the counter. Ah, Russia.

We napped on couches while awaiting our car for the airport. I awakened later to the sound of clinking glass beer bottles. The refrig was being restocked. How about that. So I bought a few bottles of beer to take home to Indiana. I couldn't find newspapers for wrapping the beer, but—remember those adult diapers? I found a new and innovative use for them.

Lori said, "Be sure you call Depends and report your discovery for their product." You read it here first: Depends Adult Diapers to protect your beer bottle shipment.

The taxi collected us for what would soon become the ride of our lives. The two of us, plus our driver and ALL our luggage was shoe-horned into the car. Lori sat in the back with backpacks. Me, in the front with our driver, whom I nicknamed Frosty because his hair had shocks the color of white-hot barbecue coals. Off we went, with Frosty accelerating quickly. Did I say that Frosty, like so many Russians we encountered, spoke no English, and he chain smoked?

"Shoulda named him Smoky," I told myself. This wasn't a public-like cab with a sign on top. It appeared to be the driver's personal car, used as a cab. I needed to lower the window down to escape the cigarette smoke so I wouldn't have to gag or suffocate. What a way to go: Survived mountain crises, but died from tobacco smoke.

We zipped along on the mountain road called the Federal Road. Maybe I got the driver's name wrong, again. Speedy would have been accurate. He seemed to handle the car well enough, and thankfully he slowed down in the one town we passed through where livestock roamed the berm of the road like a pasture. I jumped the first time he honked the horn at the cattle.

We were about 45 minutes into the four-hour drive when I noticed cars in front of us coming to a complete stop. "What's this?" I wondered. Beyond them, I spotted a 2.5 ton truck with military colors and markings being driven backward and sideways across the road. The truck came to an abrupt stop across both lanes. When we were just a few cars away from the truck, I could see inside the canvas-covered cargo area a squad of maybe 20 soldiers in combat gear carrying machine guns and wearing helmets. They jumped from the truck and took up a position further down the road from us on the other side of the truck.

Our car was positioned on the brow of a rise. Looking beyond the military truck toward a valley, I realized the highway was completely clear of traffic coming from the other direction. Not a single vehicle moved toward us. The highway stretching into the valley below looked abandoned. The road ahead was effectively blocked by the green and brown truck, with armed troops now stationed at the front and back of the truck allowing no movement—pedestrian or vehicular. Their weapons were drawn and carried waist high, at the ready.

"Not good," I said aloud. To myself, I whispered, "Whatever is going on, this looks serious."

And because we were in Russia, martial law, which is what I saw out the windshield, struck me as a time to go on personal red alert. Constitutional rights here would not go far; if any existed. Plus we were Americans in a foreign land with which the USA does not have the greatest relationship. And we didn't speak Russian. Where had I put the business card of my cousin, the woman with the State Department embassy station somewhere in Russia?

Our driver got out, making sure we clearly understand his emphatic gestures that we should keep our butts inside his car. He started making—and then taking—calls on his cell phone. Speedy could talk even faster than he drove. He paced up to the military truck and back to the car, all the while talking high-speed Russian. He listened some. Finally, after ten minutes or more, he let himself back in the car and lighted another cigarette from the one he was smoking.

I gesture to him, trying to ask what happened, asking with words saying: "What gives? What's up? What happened?" and I pointed at militia.

Getting it, Speedy-Frosty-Smoky nodded. And then he said with expression and volume—"Ka-Boom!" and lifted both his open hands, palms up.

Understanding that to mean an explosion or explosions had occurred, I grew more concerned. I spent eight years in the military, had some understanding of what bombings or rocket fire can do, knew a little about where we were in proximity to Georgia, and remembered the troops at the first ski lift. "Oh, shit!" I thought. Forgive my French.

Lori and I hadn't said much to this point. After the driver's "explosion," she started up: "What's going on? What has happened? Why do those soldiers have guns? What will we do?"

Good questions all. And since she asked, I felt she had a right to know what might be unfolding.

I said, "This may just be an annoyance. An inconvenience. On the other hand, I think given that we're near Georgia, this is some kind of civil unrest. I hope it isn't terrorism or the beginning of a civil war."

Silence from the back seat. Perhaps I said too much, in the wrong way. Then in all seriousness comes a remark that reminded me of when we were high up on the mountain and Lori confessed of "being afraid of heights." She now said: "Why'd you tell me that?" She was serious, yet it sounded funny. But I didn't laugh.

"Well, because you asked. And I thought you were entitled to know. You already beat me up some because you mistakenly thought I didn't give you all the info I had on the dangers of the mountain. So here you go—that's what I think we're looking at."

Silence followed, behind lips and a face that frowned.

Frosty/Smoky/Speedy took and received more cell calls. I expect his car had been motionless for 30 minutes now. The river alongside the roadway churned like crazy, foaming with snowmelt from the glacier. It roiled frenetically with chaotic force. I told myself, "The river is metaphor for our predicament."

The cell phone rang again. He answered, and listened for a moment. He handed me the phone and I looked at him dumbfounded, thinking, "Who do I know in Russia?"

It was Victoria, our sponsor, whom last we saw at the rental check-out. "Walter. This is Victoria. There has been explosion. There is destruction of the Federal Road."

"I understand. What are your plans for us?" I ask.

"Do not know, Walter."

"Victoria. We've been here for 30 minutes. We need to get to Mineral Vody. Now. We need to make our flight to Moscow. It will take off soon and that is the last flight today. There's little time. Get us there safely ASAP. Evacuate us by helicopter. Get on the telephone and get a chopper here to pick us up. This is an emergency. Our travel insurance will cover this," I said, hoping I understood how the evacuation clause worked in the policy.

Victoria listened and understood me, which I appreciated. She did not argue nor fiddle fart around. She said simply, "I call now."

Wishing to have some control and needing follow-up info, I said, "Call me back as soon as you find out."

Call back Victoria did. It was 15 long, long minutes which I spent praying. I couldn't tell if Lori in the back seat was crying. For support, I slid my right hand between the seat and the car door to hold her hand. Touch is what we humans thrive on. I always encourage patient's families to touch their loved ones in the hospital, most especially when they are in the active dying process. Gentle touch comforts. It says, "Security, safety." A hand provides warmth. I expected Lori needed that. And I wanted it to ensure my calmness. Right now I needed all the calmness, clarity, and confidence I had within me. "Dear God, help us," I said—maybe aloud.

Speedy's cell phone rang. He answered quickly, looked at me, and handed me the phone.

"Walter, Victoria here."

"Did you speak to the pilot?" I asked.

"I talk to pilot yes. He said, 'Russian air space, it is closed. Helicopter not possible,'" Victoria said, emotionless.

I was crushed. I'd been pinning my hopes on a rescue. Thinking it through, I realized if air space were closed here, perhaps there was a hold on all flights into and out of Mineral Vody, as it was so close by air. If that were the case, how long before the ban was lifted?

"Oh shit," I thought. "Not good." "We have a serious issue—big time," came out of my mouth.

Victoria instructed Speedy to return us to the Ozon Hotel in Terklot where we stayed. She would catch up with us and we'd talk it over further. So we turned around and headed back from where we came, leaving cars stranded in and along that section of the Federal Road as though it were a parking lot. No traffic entered the valley from the opposite direction, which told me the road, or perhaps a bridge, had been destroyed—or traffic was blocked by the military just as we were.

I prayed. I briefed Lori on what I knew for sure and said simply, "I don't know," to her questions I couldn't answer. "We should know more after we get to the hotel and talk to Victoria."

Suddenly, Speedy brought the car to a stop on the highway, across from some houses. "Oh, shit" again came to my mind and probably my lips. "What now?" We waited there, motionless. I gestured to Speedy—no response. "Oh, shit." Were we about to be handed off to terrorists? Or protectors? Victoria said nothing about this.

A girl, well a young woman, waif-like, dressed nicer than many of the peasants we'd seen, approached the car, let herself into the back seat, and sat next to Lori. She closed the door and off we zoomed. For a while I thought, "Who in the world are you?" In a moment of grace what I think to say is, "Do you speak English?"

Quietly, she said, "Yes."

"What has happened?"

She couldn't explain, or perhaps had been instructed to say nothing beyond the word: "Explosion."

There that word was again. My training as a journalist surfaced, I wanted to ask, "What exploded? Where? When? Why? How? Were there fatalities, injuries? And, "What does this mean for travelers like us?" For whatever reason, I didn't think to ask our passenger, "Who are you?"

Is it a scientific law, I think, that during an information vacuum, conjecture and misinformation flow in at light speed to fill the void. The law might go on to state that bad info seems better than no info. Well, maybe the scientific law is: Vacuums fill in. But methinks this applies to society and communication.

However, I didn't want to get tangled up in flawed thinking or fretting, so I tried to suspend judgement. I told myself: "Make no judgments and reach no conclusions. I will observe what I observe.

I will have keen awareness. I will be wary. And I will be wary of judging, of forecasting."

Speedy-Smoky-Frosty was zipping us back to the hotel with our new passenger.

Victoria checked in by telephone and said, "I will meet you later at hotel. Meantime my manager will take care of you."

"Who is your manager?" I asked.

"She sits in car with you," Victoria said.

I found it in me to laugh at myself. So important were the big questions, that I neglected to ask the obvious question to the woman getting in the car: "Who are you?" Maybe the needle on my poise and calm meter wasn't exactly where I wanted it.

Leelah, age 28, was the manager. For now, our fate rested in her hands. We would obviously miss our flight out of Mineral Vody, the last flight of the day. That meant we would also miss our connecting flight from Moscow back to the United States. Not good. I rebuked myself for not being on Jim's earlier flight. Instead of lingering at the Moscow mega-airport, we were in harm's way on the wrong side of the frontier.

At our hotel, Leelah immediately began to using the cell phone and computer to mediate on our behalf with the airlines. The hotel staff informed us we needed to re-register back in, then later reversed itself to have us check out, and would later reverse itself again to check back in. What gives, I wondered. I threw up my hands at the clerk. The clerk threw up her hands at me.

Leelah counseled me, saying simply: "Walter. Please be patient."

"Easy for you to say," I thought.

Later, when Victoria showed up, her first words were, "The road is opened now." Her plan was to move us immediately from the hotel, passing us into the darkness of night and on to Mineral Vody to overnight there.

I balked. "No. That is a bad plan Victoria. We know these people," as I pointed to the hotel staff. "We know you. And you speak English. We don't speak Russian. We are safe here. This is a refuge. We will stay here tonight and you arrange travel for us in the morning." I said all this very firmly.

To my relief, Victoria accepted this position. And she even arranged the lower outfitter's rate for us to stay, but "No," she would not pay for the room as I asked.

Switching gears, she then said, "To get airline tickets there will be penalty for new issue and it will cost you 14,000 to 15,000 ruble."

"I understand," I said, "We'll put it on my credit card."

"Not possible," Victoria said matter of factly. With sudden firm finality, she added, "You pay cash, USD (United States dollars) or ruble."

I said back, "We are almost out of both rubles and USD. We don't have that kind of cash. We need to put it on the credit card."

Her look reminded me of one I got years ago from a Franciscan nun at a Catholic elementary school who saw standing before her an impudent wet-behind-the-ears schoolboy. "Not possible, I tell you. Cash only."

I began praying and praying and praying. "We don't have that kind of cash," I restated.

Victoria: "You must pay cash. Only cash," she said, exasperated.

Before I could protest again she introduced another possibility where we might use the credit card. "Okay. We drive you to Mineral Vody tomorrow. There you buy your own tickets. You fly to Moscow. And then you get tickets there for trip to United States." And she named an airport that wasn't our airport of origin at Moscow.

"Wait a minute. That's not our airport," I protested. Our airport is Sheremetyevo in Moscow. That's where we flew into and had reservations to fly out of. We must fly from Mineralnye Vody Airport to Sheremetyveo in Moscow." And I resumed praying while I waited for her to speak.

I had just about fainted when she suggested the alternate airport. Oh, my God, Victoria was just going to arbitrarily fly us into one of Moscow's four airports and a major league mess would worsen. We'd be broke financially and at the wrong airport.

Part of my prayer was a creative way to resolve the cash shortfall position we found ourselves in. Suddenly—inspiration!

"Look," I said. "We came here in good faith. We didn't know you or your organization. We paid a lot of money in advance to you, trusting that you would do what your promotional information said you would. You did, and we appreciate that—thank you. Now, here's what I want you to do for us." And I kept praying and praying as I spoke.

Then I said: "We don't have the cash to pay for the flights now. I do have such savings available in a bank at home. I cannot get to that savings now. I cannot, you tell me, use a credit card. Therefore, what I want your organization to do is to front the rubles to us. Then when we get home, I will repay this money. Due to circumstances beyond our control—the explosion—we find ourselves in this predicament. This is not our fault."

"Not possible," Victoria said, parroting Russia's answer for too many circumstances.

"We need some consideration here," I said firmly. And I prayed and prayed.

Victoria: "Not possible."

"Why?" I asked.

Maybe I was tone deaf to her answer; Maybe I didn't hear it. Maybe I didn't need to. Whatever she said, here's what I did.

I am long a believer that if someone can't help me, or refuses to help me with a pressing problem, I should ask to speak with their supervisor. I do so in hopes that the additional consideration will lead to an over-rule of what the subordinate told me. So I did just that with Victoria. "Then, I need to talk to your boss. Now," I said firmly.

"Not possible—I no can do that," she said.

With some impatience and I expect more volume than normal in my voice, I exclaimed to Victoria: "Call somebody and ask!" I don't think I was shouting, but my voice surely sounded louder to my ears. Quietly and fervently, I prayed and prayed.

"Hokay. I call accountant," Victoria said, relenting from her position of "not possible."

Lori, for the most part, had deferred to me on this negotiation. She tried to interject a time or two some words that softened, weakened, my position. Undiplomatic, insensitive, and maybe slightly arrogant, I lightly stepped on her foot two different times. Lori, like me, is a gentle spirit. But I know there are times for firmness, where you absolutely need to man up to someone. And in certain circumstances you need to do so immediately, or you won't ever have a second chance. This was one of those times. We only needed one voice, and that voice needed to be resolute, not kind; even a little demanding and expectant. Later, thankfully, Lori accepted my apology.

Victoria told us to wait. I prayed more, and asked Lori to pray also.

When Victoria returned from calling the accountant, she simply announced, "Accountant he say 'Hokay.' We advance you rubles."

How this happened I didn't ask and I still don't need to know. I do know that a while later the rubles arrived.

Thank you, God of mercies!

Praise the Lord.

And rock and roll.

Leelah and Victoria teamed up, made calls to the airlines, and paved the way for tickets for us to fly from Mineralnye Vody to Sheremetyevo, the correct Moscow airport. They also called Delta, our carrier from Moscow to the USA, explained the problem and told them we would not be on our pre-arranged flight that evening from Moscow to the USA, due to extenuating circumstances.

Finally, after a delivery to Victoria at the hotel, she came to me and counted out 15,000 rubles. Oh my word. Praise the Lord indeed!

We had accomplished a lot since the "explosion" happened in early afternoon. Darkness had fallen by the time we concluded our business with Victoria and Leelah. I sincerely thanked Victoria and asked if I might give her a hug. She complied, but it was a distant hug. Nonetheless, I was happy to give it. But these Russians— oh, man. Of course, I probably violated cultural protocol and left Victoria thinking, "Those crazy Americans."

We had a chance before Victoria's arrival to get something to eat. Wally Berg, the international travel guide we'd met earlier, was in the dining room. He sought to dispel worries, calling what happened, in my words, "a hiccup," and predicted that normalcy would soon be restored. Would that that Wally Berg was right and Wally Glover and Lori soon would be safe at home. Lori certainly had been a trooper throughout this difficulty.

The dinner entrée was fish heads again. Oh, geez ma neez. I think we ate rice and soup. Lori and I are both emotionally spent, weary, and I will allow—worried. Georgia lay just over the mountains. Was the "explosion" (whatever it was and whatever it meant) an isolated incident? "Dear God, that this isn't the beginning of a civil war."

Wait! No, they wouldn't have re-opened the road if fighting had broken out. And obviously air space was re-opened because they are booking reservations and the airport is open. Crisis averted? Crisis looming? I resumed prayers of both gratitude, and of petition to get us safely home.

Monday, June 28, 2010

My sleep was restless, but thankfully I got some. I awakened at 5 a.m. and showered. Shortly afterward, Lori did the same. We ate in the dining room and waited at the hotel's front door like kids watching for a school bus. Our luggage sat on the porch. The telephone rang at the front desk, which in the early morning was unattended. I headed over that way and Lori said, "You're not going to answer that are you?"

"Yep," I said. I had a feeling this call might be intended for us.

As I suspected, the caller was Victoria. Meantime Lori advised our ride had arrived, which I told Victoria. She asked who was minding the store and I reported there was no one at the registration desk. I was supposed to be given an invoice to sign for the rubles, but no invoice and no one to ask. Her "Hokay" sounded more like, "Not okay," but we said "goodbye" because the taxi was waiting.

We loaded our bags in a driving rain and zipped away—until the driver stopped the car at the hotel gate house. "What now?" I wondered. Luckily, the stop was just a courtesy for our driver to greet the gatekeeper who was on duty yesterday. We too exchanged a wave with him. Of course the driver didn't speak English, but did chain smoke cigarettes. Like yesterday's car, this appeared to be the driver's personal vehicle. As the day before, we moved along at a good clip. The rain slackened, and then stopped. As we passed through small villages, we watched peasant Russians walk to their jobs and students in uniforms carrying books to school. Other cars were on the road, but everything in front soon moved behind us because our driver knew only one speed: fast. He also was safe, handling the car well and not reckless.

I thought I recognized the trouble point where we were stopped the day before, but maybe not. I watched the river, still roiling and frothing, fueled by glacier and snow melt in these lower elevations and making its way who knows where. I thought perhaps the rivers would flow to the Black or Caspian seas. Unlike Africa, I didn't see anyone carrying water in jugs on their heads, so I presumed wells were dug hereabouts; Maybe not. Maybe the villagers and townspeople depended on the river for drinking, cooking, and washing. The things we Americans take for granted.

The sun chased away the clouds. Blue sky cheered me up. And the driver sped onward. Oh, no! Suddenly, without warning, the driver turned abruptly off the main road. What now? Where now? He said something, looking at Lori in the rear view mirror, she sitting in the back seat, and then he looked at me.

I got it. I hoped we were going to Victoria's office or house or something. She surely wouldn't let us leave the country without signing an invoice, or some kind of affidavit that we owed money. And in a few minutes the driver pulled the vehicle up to a collection of ramshackle buildings and motioned for us to wait in the car. A few minutes passed and he returned with a form indicating the need for my signature. I didn't read Russian but I could read 15000 rubles. I signed—gladly. He returned inside and then returned to the car, handing me a document, first opening it for me to read. It was a kind of announcement with a seal. Victoria, God love her, provided paperwork to document the "Explosion on Federal Road." This would become key evidence with the airlines, and on getting back home with the travel insurance company. Thank you Victoria, God bless you.

I don't know exactly how fast we travelled, but I do know what the scenery looks like when I drive 70 miles an hour on Interstate 65 going to and from my hospital ministries in Bedford and Salem. We passed the scenery considerably faster than 70 miles an hour on I-65. Finally, the driver slowed to a crawl in an area of open road. "What now" I thought again and maybe even said aloud, "Holy shit!" I think this I did say that aloud.

Once again military vehicles occupied the road ahead, plus a platoon of combat outfitted men with guns at the ready. The driver reached back and fastened his seat belt. Wanting Lori to stay calm, and wanting me to stay calm too, I passed my right hand back to hold hers. As we approached I saw what I'd call a checkpoint, except traffic continued in both directions at a slow speed, but the cars were not being stopped. We cleared the area in an orderly fashion and the driver said, "Hokay."

"Thank you, God for travel mercies today," I thought. This happened two more times before we reached the airport. Each time my heart rate increased. Thank you also to my prayer warriors at home for safety and travel mercies.

A couple of hours into what was customarily a four hour drive, the driver smoked his last cigarette from the pack. On checking around the car he must have realized he was out. At his stop in the next village I knew what was coming. He pulled in at a small grocery store with cigarette signs. Yep, he needed more smokes. He looked at us and gestured clearly to see if we wanted drinks, sodas. We said "No," shaking our heads. The driver must have read our minds around being broke, or maybe Victoria had told him about us. When he came out of the store with cigarettes, he also carried two cold drinks. He put one in each of our hands and smiled. Then, he lit a cigarette, took a deep drag, and our drag race resumed. The sun shone brilliantly now and the temperature grew warmer. We thanked him and drank our sodas.

In less three hours (a speed record to go with Sergey's, I presumed), we approached Mineral Vody and signs for the airport The driver pulled off the side of road, no military or police in sight. I felt unworried, but curious. The driver's skill, coolness, and compassion toward us gave me confidence in him. Later, I assigned this man hero status for his conduct as our advocate at the airport. As the car came to a stop, he reached under his seat and pulled out a kind of billfold. From it, he pulled a large, multi-colored rectangular ruble. "Never saw a ruble like that," I told myself, noting its colors. He tucked it up behind the sun visor, replaced his billfold to safe keeping, and off we went. I wondered. It was three hours on the dot when we pulled up to the airport security gate.

But we did not go through the gate. We turned left down a dirt road maybe 50 meters before the checkpoint, where vehicles lined up and where I saw drivers and passengers answering questions and having their passports reviewed. Our driver stopped the car on this side road near a building and we waited. Then, one large officer, maybe military, maybe civilian police, approached our car. His sidearm was holstered at his waist. He came up to my door and said, "Passports." This was a huge man—even his hat and its badge were large. As I reached into my pocket for both our passports, our driver left the car. I handed the officer both our passports. What happened next I didn't see, but Lori from the backseat clearly saw what happened. The driver walked to where the officer stood, in clear view of Lori's window.

"The driver handed him a funny colored ruble thing," she told me later. The officer conducted a few seconds' inspection of our passports. The driver returned to the car and relaxed behind the steering wheel. Our passports were returned through the car window to me. The driver then started the car and continued down the side road, made a turn here and there, and soon parked the car within a block of the front door of Mineralnye Vody Airport. Did we observe bribery, or was this the accepted way of conducting business in Russia?

We walked to a baggage security checkpoint inside the airport and found no one in front of us; odd, as we were accustomed to waiting. Our driver stayed right with us—also strange, as he would normally leave after dropping us at the airport. Lori's luggage cleared without incident. When the bag checker reached into my bag, and held up one of the adult diaper wrapped beers and said something that sounded like a question.

In English, I responded, "Glass, breakable." She seemed to understand and accepted that. Then she held up one of my water bottles with a built in filtering system. To her, it probably resembled a Molotov cocktail or bomb with a short aluminum fuse-like drinking spout sticking out the top. However, the bottle was empty and plastic. The checker looked at me inquisitively and said something in Russian. I gestured as if holding it and drinking. She accepted this pantomime answer. We cleared baggage inspection and moved to the ticket counter. Our driver, who was about to become a saint, stayed with us.

The driver asked for our passports and began talking with the ticket agent, a woman behind the counter. Her work area had bars in front of the space separating her from passengers, and our driver. Hmmm. She was a big woman—not as large as the checkpoint soldier/policeman, but portly and buxom. I soon named her Ms. Buxom. The driver held our passports in front of her and they talked. Soon their conversation increased in decibel level, accompanied by gestures. Although I couldn't understand the Russian words, it became clear, as our driver occasionally gestured our way, that he was lobbying for us. Had Victoria coached him on something? The so-called dialogue broke down, and he motioned me forward before Ms. Buxom and threw up his hands. I smiled to myself, thinking, "You are doing a good impression of me." The driver walked behind Lori and stood fast, glaring at Ms. Buxom. He was physically standing with us—a show of support I appreciated.

A stern-looking Ms. Buxom with hair knotted in a tightly braided bun behind a face that looked like it had swallowed prunes a minute ago now addressed herself to me, in Russian of course.

I immediately called a halt and said "Translator. English translator." Buxom understood immediately and called her own halt to matters. A few minutes went by and up came a slight, fairly attractive young woman with straight blonde hair dressed in a blue business suit. Consistent with the "B" alliteration, I dubbed the translator Ms. Blondie because she was. She addressed me in English and I simply said "We are checking in for the flight to Moscow Sheremetyevo Airport." I showed her our passports and added, "It has been arranged."

Ms. Blondie presented the passports to Ms. Buxom, who had already apparently pulled up our names on a passenger manifest. The issue between she and the translator became clear. Buxom spoke to Blondie, pointing to the names on our passports, and the screen. Blondie spoke back to Buxom, and Buxom replied to Blondie.

Ms. Blondie turned to me and said business-like, "Your tickets are ready and the cost is 16,000 rubles."

This price was above the 14,000 rubles the tickets were supposed to cost, according to Victoria. Victoria and I had agreed to an extra 1,000 rubles for expenses. Thus, we were carrying 15.000 rubles, plus a few personal miscellaneous small bills in both rubles and USD. Suddenly the tickets were 16,000 rubles. Oh, geez—a 2,000 ruble increase.

"No, that's wrong," I said. "Our tickets cost 14,000 rubles. This transaction was arranged last night and the price clearly was listed and agreed to at 14,000 rubles." I realized I carried no paperwork to support my position. Oh, no.

Blondie turned to Buxom and they conversed in Russia. Buxom spoke, then Blondie. Again, Blondie turned to me and said, "The tickets they cost rubles 16,000."

I held my ground. "No they don't. They cost 14,000 rubles. I have 14,000 rubles and I am prepared to pay that (patting my backside where my billfold was). Then I began praying and praying and praying. Lori got the drift and began talking to Blondie in a kind way. As before, I lightly stepped on her foot. This was no time for gentleness, and we really needed only one spokesperson.

"Tell her they cost 14,000 rubles" I said to Blondie nodding to Buxom. Back and forth went Blondie and Buxom. Blondie turned to me and gave some remarkable new information. "Fourteen thousand rubles was yesterday's price, and it was for the late flight, not this one."

In Indiana you might characterize such information by saying, "I smell a rat." I kept praying and praying. I pointedly glared at Buxom. I sensed she was driving what I now believe to be an extortion and Blondie was complicit. I said to Blondie, "We are not being treated fairly. Airlines don't change prices like that." And I pray again.

She passed this info to Buxom who sternly said something back.

Blondie: "Well that is the way it is," she said with an air of finality.

As is said in the Bible of some of its heroes and heroines, I stood firm. I repeated my position word for word as I had just stated it. "We are not being treated fairly." I glared at both the women. I prayed. And my action step was to take from my billfold 14,000 rubles and place them on the counter under the jail-like bars before Buxom.

What would be a graced exchange followed between the B and B twins, in Russian of course. I'd love to know what they said. What I heard next might just as well have been, "Your prayer was answered."

Ms. Blondie looked at me and said: "Airline change mind. Price for you for this flight now is 14,000 rubles."

Praise the Lord!

I did not act smug, arrogant, or in their faces. Was this an attempt at extortion? I don't need to judge it. In the end fairness was upheld.

I conducted business, paying 14,000 rubles to Buxom for our two tickets for the next flight from Mineralyne Vody to our airport of origin in Russia. I had Blondie confirm this, looking at our tickets, which she did.

Our driver, God bless this man whom I nominated for sainthood, still remained unwaveringly with us. He clearly understood what transpired when the money exchanged hands, and he would have understood the Russian side of the exchange. I gave Saint Driver a huge bear hug. Unfortunately, I couldn't give him a big tip for his driving, his companionship, advocacy, and compassion. But I tell you this, and I hope my words get back to you Saint Driver. I still pray for you when I see the poster of Elbrus on my kitchen wall.

Lori and I said goodbye to our driver, expressing gratitude and God's blessings to him. I then asked Ms. Blondie if I might give her a hug. "Yes, do so," she said bashfully. Since I seemed to be on a roll, I asked her to help us negotiate the baggage check-in. She even helped us carry our bags, nodded to someone, and suddenly we were in the front of the line which made Lori terribly uncomfortable for having jumped the que. Maybe I should have felt badly too, but I was more than ready to reach the gate and depart.

But first I used the restroom, which necessitated a trip past Ms. Buxom's cube. She was there and did not have a customer, so I made eye contact with her and gave her a Namaste bow I learned at Everest. Hands clasped before my chest, I bowed low to her, saying the words I learned: "The Divine in me greets the Divine in you." When used with Tibetan Buddhists and some other faith practitioners, this greeting generates a return bow with the same words. The greeting recognizes that divinity resides within each of the speakers. Ms. Buxom smiled—yes, she smiled at me. Yes, at me! And she returned my bow. How about that for closure!

My next blessing came when I entered a restroom that was fairly clean. Thanks, God.

We had a nice visit at our gate with a Russian MD who lived near Las Vegas in Henderson, NV, where my young friend Kylee Thomas lived at the time. I often skied with Kylee, her brother Ian, and their dad Steve Thomas, my good friend from Columbus, with Dick Vance at Telluride. The physician worked in organ transplant research at UNLV. Hearing that he and his wife had lost a child, I used my pastoral counsel skills to hopefully give him some solace. He was grateful.

We boarded our plane and headed for Moscow, in air leg one of our homeward trip. As we neared Moscow's huge Sheremetyevo Airport, I contemplated the next steps: Retrieve our bags, and then connect with Delta Airlines to arrange our flight home. Plus, our families needed to know we were okay. For now, all they knew was that we didn't arrive on time and were not where we were supposed to be—back home again in Indiana. Then, we needed something to eat, to liquidate our few rubles for dollars, and find chairs to sleep in. During all this, we would push the luggage before us in a three wheeled cart. That was the plan I conceived.

Little did I know, the airline difficulties would resume, Moscow style. Things began innocently enough, except now we were sufficiently shell shocked that all manner of travel innocence was long gone. The pilot announced our approach to landing in Moscow, and then we circled. And we circled. And we circled, with Moscow clearly in sight below us. No advisory came from the pilot over the PA. We continued to circle. Was there a lot of air traffic that needed to clear? Were they having a security problem on the ground?

When finally we landed and taxied to our gate, the buzz began among the passengers. Maybe it was a rumor on the flight, maybe it was an overheard conversation, maybe this was somehow observable to someone in the know. But the understanding some passengers spoke of as we deplaned was that all arriving flights had been waved off, effectively suspended from landing for a while. An English speaking voice said, "The airport was shut down."

We never knew for sure what caused the delay. I just prayed the events along the Federal Road through the mountains hadn't carried over to Moscow. It wasn't funny to consider the World War II military assault called Operation Barbarosa that crossed through the Elbrus Territory had advanced all the way east and laid siege to Moscow. I had prayed fervently, "Dear God, do not let history repeat itself. Not now." After we landed, I prayed in thanksgiving tagging on an earnest postscript: "God, speed us to the USA."

We claimed our bags and headed to the Delta Airlines desk to arrange travel for the next day. But, as I said earlier, "Nothing is easy in Russia." Things we take for granted in the USA are damnably difficult. The Delta office at the airport had closed for the day. "What?" I yelled at the recorded message. "Unbelievable! Did they take the day off? You don't believe in religion here and besides it isn't even Sunday." I was fuming. We wanted to book a flight for the next day, but no one was there to arrange it. "Day off . . . day of rest. Cripes! This is Monday."

Thanks to Lori's persistence and the information desk woman's patience with Lori's gentle way (as opposed to my searing brusqueness), we somehow found a live voice to speak with at Delta.

The call started off great, "Ah, yes, Mr. Glover, we've been expecting your call. Your sponsor notified us of your problem."

I explained we were overdue at home and wished to book a flight for the next day.

"Ah, well that will not be possible. Tomorrow, Tuesday, all the flights from Moscow to JFK are full. So sorry. In fact that is the case for several days. We suggest your party find a nice hotel, make plans to visit Moscow and see the sights for the next two to three days. Then we can get you out at the end of the week when we have an opening."

You know the drill by now—I started praying.

I tried to keep Lori updated on the conversation as it happened. "Ask for standby," she said.

I did so.

"There is no standby or wait list," he said.

Lori snapped a frown at this information.

"How about business/first class?" I asked

"Yes, I can put the two of you in first class," he said.

"What will that cost?"

"That will be $3000." And he paused perhaps for effect, and added, "$3000 each."

Having learned some Russian by now, I said, "Not possible." I wanted to say yes, but knew that substantially exceeded what our insurance would pay. I kept praying and praying.

A ray of insight visited me. I tried to prick the dude's conscience by asking, "What happened to our seats on yesterday's flight? Were they turned a second time, and resold at the last minute at a huge profit to Delta?" I heard my voice turn accusing. He said he had no information on that.

A grace followed my mean-spiritedness. I grew calm and asked, "Delta is a part of the affiliated Sky Partners group or whatever you call it, right?

"Yes, we are members."

"Work this problem backward from the United States. We don't need to fly into JFK at New York City. We don't need to fly into New Jersey. Work it backward from the airports in the states with your partners and tell me what you can do. Find our flight that way. Reverse the process."

And now I was *really* praying.

After a few minutes of research while we waited, the clerk said: "Mr. Glover, I have done what you asked. Yes, we can fly you from Moscow to Atlanta and then to Indianapolis, the both of you, tomorrow morning. Is that acceptable?"

Remembering the $3,000 first class seats, I asked, "How much?"

"For $300, each."

"$300 each I heard you say. Correct?"

"Yes," he responded.

"We'll take it!" I jubilantly exclaimed, "Thank you, Jesus!" What great news. Lori and I were smiling like we won the lottery as I found out where and when to collect the tickets.

Lori reached her family in Indianapolis by telephone and provided an update. They were relieved, to say the least. I left a message for son Dominic. These calls were a challenge as we had to find where to buy phone cards, then locate a place to use them. Again, the things we Americans take for granted. Before the calls, all our family at home knew was: a) we didn't show in Indiana when we were supposed to return; b) we were somewhere in Russia, and c) our exact location was a mystery.

I learned it takes a while to climb not one, but two, Russian mountains. And these events confirmed for me that fervent prayer is an antidote to conundrums.

Our tasks accomplished, we looked for a place to spend our few remaining rubles and USD to eat. We were both thinking red-white-and-blue, so Lori chose a TGIF knock-off place with local touches. Our Russian waiter was named Stas, a nice young man. A soccer game played on television—the World Cup, so the place was crowded and deafening. To slake my appetite in this Russian restaurant I ordered a cheeseburger and fries, and Lori got some kind of chicken melt and a huge green salad. Plus a couple of German beers, and another one, to split; Alas no USA brews on the menu. The food tasted great!

Then we window shopped, while pushing our luggage on a cart like homeless people. For safekeeping, we didn't check our luggage, but kept it with us at all times. We window shopped without buying: Rubleless and almost penniless. Homeless? Not quite.

We sought shuteye on couches in Terminal F near the area where we slept on the way in. This time, we joined other airport urchins awaiting flights. Airport Security rousted us. What was acceptable going to the mountain, was no longer allowed—or so it seemed. "Dear God, don't let me become jaded." I thought.

Like refugees from the World War II's invasion of Moscow, we moved with our luggage, seeking shelter elsewhere. Our next squatter's area must have been acceptable to Security. Lori quickly fell asleep in an upholstered chair across from me, with our luggage on the cart between us.

We felt a bit like homeless people. More accurately stated, we were people with a homeland who wandered afar. We held the hope and promise of a paper passport. And, drumroll, we held more paper airline tickets that didn't cost an arm and leg. We had little currency to speak of, but our Homecoming with a capital "H," drew closer with each tick of the clock.

Tuesday, June 29, 2010

I awakened in our "refugee camp" at 4:30 a.m. Our foot soldier security guy was making rounds, as he did all during the night. He now saw that, for comfort, I propped my foot atop the container of an artificial potted plant. The security guy who earlier made rounds without so much as a peep, said something Russian and pointed at my foot. I moved it, and to myself said, "Teehee, this is a demonstration by Officer Control." To myself, I called him a bully. But, no matter. This was his turf and I was a visitor, an expatriate soon to be home. I would roll with it. This was his home court.

Lori and I took turns visiting a nearby bathroom and minding the bags. The restroom was clean, with hot water that was actually hot—more good fortune. Lori was in fairly good spirits. I felt sore all over from sleeping in a chair, but had much to be chipper about—today we would leave for home. Hooray and praise the Lord! We window shopped the closed stores until Starbucks—a Lori favorite, opened for business. We treated ourselves to warm muffins and great java, plus their seats felt comfy to my all-over soreness. We looked a little out of place with our luggage cart, but I found an out-of-the-way corner in Starbucks to park it.

The custom at Starbucks is for waitresses to write the customer's name on the cups to ensure accurate delivery. I asked them to also write our names in Russian, which they delighted in doing. I still have my cup, and Lori's, atop the frig. We paid in a combo of rubles and dollars, as I remember.

We secured our plane tickets from Delta without issue, checked our bags, cleared security, and wait-wait-waited at the gate. Finally we boarded our plane, and pushed back from the gate. We taxied and were soon airborne, out of Russia to Atlanta, Georgia, US of A. Thank you, God.

Count 'em...62 hours after leaving the mountain, finally we were going home.

It seems that, while in Russia, Lori and I climbed not one mountain, but two. The second one—getting out of the country—may have been the more difficult. Considering we didn't train for the second challenge as we did for Mt. Elbrus, I think we did well on mountain number two. Who trains for that? Prayer certainly helped. And grace.

At last, we landed in Atlanta. Thank you, God: The USA! Passport Control and Customs at Atlanta went seamlessly. After a short wait we boarded another Delta jet and were one nap away from home.

We touched down at Indy on 29 June, 2010. Mystically from the sky or the cornfields, if you heard someone singing "Back Home Again in Indiana" that evening, it was me. Later I heard the Beatles' oldie "Back In the USSR" and its refrain, "Oh, how happy we are," live at Cool Creek Park in Indy with Lori. Several weeks later I heard the Beatles sing it again while riding in a van playing on a CD as friends and I re-entered the United States from Canada. I used to like that Beatles song and its refrain. I never bother singing it any more.

POSTSCRIPT

Over the next several months Lori and I would transition from colleagues and climbers of Elbrus to become a couple, and then grow to be life partners—soulmates. We each wore a ring fashioned around small pieces of Elbrus stones we collected the morning we departed from Barrel 7. Each ring has the shape of Elbrus inscribed on it.

January, 2017 – Elbrus Epilogue

Our relationship was joyfully launched in earnest during the year after Elbrus. We were blessed with laughter, smiles, cooking and eating, tennis and trekking exercise, bicycling, fun with friends, visiting 80ish-year old dear Mary across the alley, concert-goings, Mass and church services, antics with grandchildren, and being in love.

After St. Vincent Peyton Manning Children's Hospital eliminated her youth obesity program and her job—arrgh—Lori spent much of the year in Colorado. She was one of 1,000 men and women cut adrift including a team of vice presidents at St. Vincent Indianapolis. Even one of my southern Indiana CEOs lost his job. When a near-30 hospital system misses budget forecasts dramatically, everyone from the executive to the environmental services housekeeper is vulnerable—across all the hospitals from impoverished small town hospital ministries to large tertiary care centers in urban areas. So Lori joined the prestigious Colorado Children's Hospital in suburban Denver. Retired, I visited for Christmas 2013, and again in 2014. We blossomed as a couple.

In the summer of 2014 she made the move to a large pediatric private practice in my town of Columbus. We were really and finally together—and a few weeks later apart, for good reason: I left for Spain and the 490 mile trek called El Camino, The Way of

St. James, still raising money for rural southern Indiana St. Vincent hospitals to combat youth obesity. Unlike St. Vincent Peyton Manning, they continued the ministry to overweight youth. When I returned from Spain a month later, we were blissfully together—a love story being lived.

Sadly, Lori later found she was not as happy as she expected, wanted, and said she needed. As the Russian mountain Elbrus had brought us together, it farewelled us apart. On the anniversary date of our summit six years before, she announced unceremoniously that she was leaving. Silly me, stupid head, I thought we were leaving together to play tennis as we had so frequently and happily done. She was leaving alright, by herself (well she took the dog). She went out the door and moved to Indianapolis. Weeks later, she landed a job there.

The issues I thought we'd resolved were not. Despite staying in touch for weeks and sharing the dog Sierra Nevada we both loved, we couldn't finish what we started in Russia and accomplish a third climb. The third climb, our personal mountain, went charmless. Lori was gone, along with Sierra.

What bereft widows and widowers teach me in grief groups around loneliness, I now suffered. Differently to be sure, as the one I had loved still lived. "Grief is the price we pay for having loved," says my mentor Alan Wolfelt Ph.D. "The groundlessness of suffering—hold it close. It will instruct you," say the Buddhists.

As I finish this Epilogue, I still wear my mountain ring from Russia. Elbrus was the gateway to a love story. And to loss.

Yet as I write these last lines, unexplored territory lies ahead: More mountains to climb, and trek training is underway for the next elevated boundary. A frontier in South America, the Peruvian sacred geologic beauty Rainbow Mountain, awaits me this May.

And I will be raising money for the Columbus Foundation for Youth, a consortium of children's agencies and wellness programs in my home community. Promise and hope are in the thin air up high, again. Thank you, God: For what was, what is, and what will be.

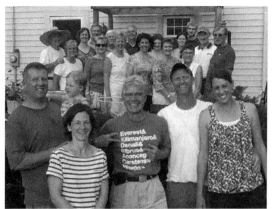

*Pre-departure farewellin party with family
and friends*

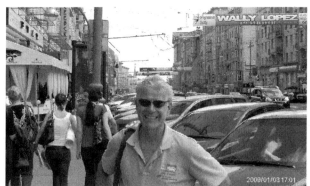

Wally meets Wally Lopez—downtown Moscow

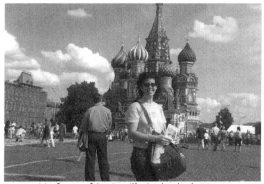

*Lori in front of St. Basil's Cathedral, Moscow,
Red Square*

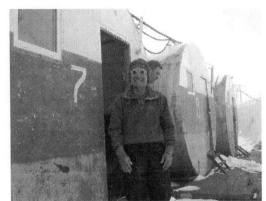

Walter at Barrel 7. Fellow climber James in background.

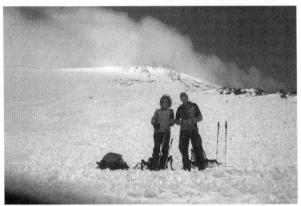

Sergey and Lori on acclimatizing hike high Mt. Elbrus

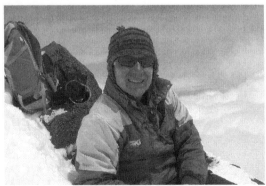

Walter in the clouds—lunch break below the summit

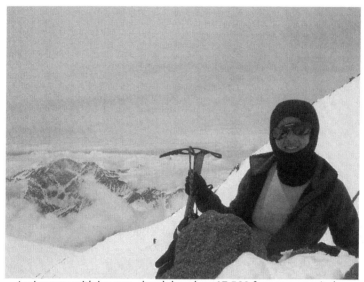

Lori secure with ice axe—lunch break at 17,500 feet on summit day

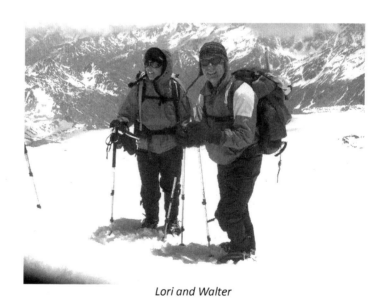

Lori and Walter

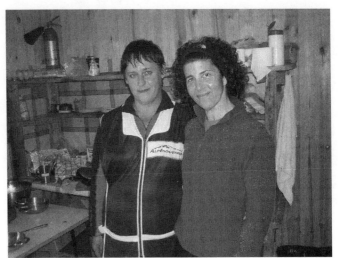

LeeAnna and Lori

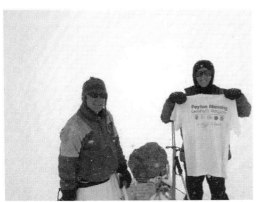

*Lori hoists Peyton Manning Children's Hospital
T-shirt to record elevation*

SECTION TWO: Mount Kosciuszko

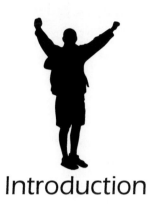

Introduction

Mount Kosciuszko in Australia, nicknamed Kozzie, was the lowest mountain I climbed on, at only 7,310 feet high. Though the challenge was small, comparatively speaking, this mountain located in the land down under somehow generated the single most revenue for 2 Trek 4 Kids, the youth obesity management, prevention, and treatment programs my climbs financially supported. Kozzie alone raised more than $26,000.

I was 63 years old when I climbed it and would turn 64 the following month. My trip "down under," as Australia is known, was in January 2011, exactly 12 months before I would head for Argentina and the tallest mountain in my sights—15,500 feet higher than Kozzie, to be exact. The Aussie trip was only a single day's climb, really an uphill walk. Twelve months later in Argentina, I wished I had reversed the order and been a year younger on the tallest mountain I would ever attempt.

The Australia trek also differed from others in that I didn't join a group. I went solo, on my own, for 12 days. This Kozzie was a one day trek, maybe two, if I chose to acclimatize. I was in a national park with the route clearly marked—no guide or climbing mates needed. Another difference—this mountain began my efforts to raise money for St. Vincent Salem and St. Vincent Dunn in Bedford as they embarked on youth weight management programs. The previous climbs in Africa and Russia raised close to $50,000 for the youth obesity program at St. Vincent Jennings in North Vernon. After start-up expenses, the money was used to scholarship kids through the clinic program.

My departure weight was 160 pounds, a little below my high school weight. After my climb with Lori in Russia, I wondered if climbing up and into a crater on the moon might be anticlimactic. And Elbrus came after climbing on two of the best known mountains in the world—to Everest Base Camp and to the summit of Kilimanjaro. It would take something epic to top all three.

Although Kozzie in Australia was a modest to mild challenge, the climb had its own singular beauty and memorable experiences. As for objective dangers, there were none. Deadly spiders were perhaps the only real danger, and if I saw one of those creatures, I didn't recognize it. So please don't expect peril, intrigue, suspense, and danger as you read on. Know, however, that to pursue a quest means you tag all its bases—well, tops—and Kozzie was on my Seven Summits list. It was, after all, a walk in the park—the Mount Kozzie National Park.

Wednesday, January 12, 2011

On the morning of my departure, I read from the book of Sirach first thing. The Catholic translation of the Bible includes Sirach and other books that didn't survive Reformation translations. I checked out the author's words concerning Elohim, the Creator God, as God unfolds the planet Earth at creation time. As Sirach says, "No words can do it justice." I hoped Sirach passages would give me a greater appreciation of what I would see down under.

Lori drove me to Indianapolis International Airport and I found myself experiencing a re-occurring lump in my throat, knowing I would be away—a long way away—for 12 days. We were together on the Russian mountain Elbrus' summit six months earlier and we both wished she could accompany me for the Down Under Expedition. She dropped me off curbside at the airport and we embraced. Goodbyes are always hard.

Lori and I climbed Mount Elbrus in Russia as business colleagues. Since then we became, the Aussies say, *mates*. We were romantically involved. Youth obesity and then mountains climbs brought us together, and soon we were exploring our future together.

I gathered my expedition bag and carry-on. I wore my backpack. And just like that, I was on my way to my fourth of the Seven Summits. I pinched myself to believe all this was happening. In spring 2007, I trekked to Mount Everest Base Camp in Nepal; In summer 2009, I climbed and stood atop Mount Kilimanjaro in Africa; six months ago Lori and I tagged the summit of Mount Elbrus in a suspense-filled time in Russia; and I headed to Mount Kozzie in Australia in January, 2011.

How improbable it all seemed—me, a kid from a small town in the flatlands of Indiana, going to world-class mountains. I grew up a "stonecutter," the nickname for our high school athletic teams, reflecting the limestone industry in our area. Piles of quarried stone blocks ringed the little community of Bedford in southern Indiana. Other than the low, rolling terrain around Bedford, I knew nothing of mountains or mountaineers while growing up. I didn't see a real mountain until I was an adult. Until then, our upland terrain and piles of limestone blocks served as my high points.

But I did have a capacity to dream, and I longed to see new places. Perhaps my wanderlust came from ancestors on the shores of Italy. In the early 1900s, my maternal immigrant family boarded shipping vessels for United States' shores. After an ocean voyage in the below water level hold of a ship, in quarters suitable for cattle, they glimpsed the Statue of Liberty. Months later they saw Victory Monument on the downtown circle of Indianapolis. Artisans in stone, they created monuments from building stone tediously quarried out of the rich limestone veins of southern Indiana. Their masterful works stretched from Washington D.C. up the northeastern corridor to Wall Street. They literally carved their future in stone, contemporary Michaelangelos. Those who didn't carve, cut the stone to size. They left behind monumental works, including the Empire State Building—and the piles of limestone rocks I climbed as a kid.

And then my dad boarded ships belonging to the United States Navy and sailed away to the Pacific Theater of World War II, helping keep me and my family and America's citizens and shores, safe.

Speaking of my dad, a relative wrote me just before my Everest expedition and said: "He certainly was adventuresome, widely-traveled, and world curious." My paternal cousin Karl Schilling said of my father, "His heritage is firmly imprinted in you." So it seemed international travel was part of my DNA from both sides of my family.

Would I indeed be able to climb on all of the Seven Summits? Such an achievement seemed unlikely, though I intended to try. When asked by the news media, or at one of my presentations to the public, "Can you do it—all seven?" I'd laugh and demur, saying: "It's crazy to think I can do it. I'm almost 65 years old. It's crazy to think a senior citizen flatlander clergy guy from the cornfields of Indiana can climb the Seven Summits."

Making these statements took the pressure off. I would add, "Of course the oldest guy to climb Everest was 80 when he did so, and the oldest guy to climb the Seven Summits was 75. So I'm still young by those standards." And then I'd laugh. I didn't wish to be immodest, but I had been around long enough to know that if I didn't believe in myself and portray confidence and poise, no one else would believe in me either.

So, there I was at the Indianapolis airport again, this time on my way to Australia. The airline self-serve check-in kiosk had konked out, so an airline ticket agent helped me. Noticing my itinerary and departure times he volunteered: "No need to wait. Let's get you on your way. Your itinerary transfer is a little tight in Chicago, we need to get you going." He set me up with an earlier departure—the first of countless kindnesses I would be accorded on this expedition. I thanked him for his initiative and added, "Bless you."

He beamed a smile back.

At the gate I found a seat and removed my backpack. As with all my climbs, the pack featured an 8 by 12 inch poster showing the mountain I was headed to, naming my hospital ministries, and that my trek would raise money for youth obesity programs. Each poster included Psalm 46:10, a favorite of mine from the Old Testament: "Be still and know that I am God." A line at the bottom of the poster instructed: *Ask this trekker for more info*. You'd be astonished how that invitation started conversations, which was the whole point.

Indeed, the couple seated next to me saw the poster and chatted me up. They were from Brisbane, Australia. We talked until boarding time and I told them that, in addition to the mountain, I intended to visit Sydney and climb its iconic Harbour Bridge, then visit the Australian Open Grand Slam Tennis Championship event. They were full of suggestions and gave me their business cards, urging me to call if I had any problems; another kindness right on the heels of the first. This husband and wife were in Indy for the International Archery Show and owned Australia's largest archery company. They warned me about the serious flooding in Australia—something I was aware of from the news, including the fact that flooding fringe areas would be part of my travel circuit.

Lori and I exchanged text messages and a brief call. I used my St. Vincent Blackberry to check the 2trek4kids.org website and found several new messages wishing me well. I said a thank you prayer to God for my loved one, my beloved family, my friends, and the 2Trek4Kids supporters.

At the first stop in Chicago, I spotted a man wearing a green Top of the World, Nepal T-shirt with a picture of the majestic Mount Everest. Hmmm. I had a shirt exactly like it at home, which is what I said to the guy. We talked shop for a minute. Like me, he had trekked to Everest Base Camp at 17,600. He climbed higher than me at 18,200 on Kala Patar, a mountain next door to Base Camp. I had to pass on Kala Patar because of acute mountain sickness and additional issues. Both of us had climbed and summited Kilimanjaro. Elbrus was on his list, so he wanted to know my impressions of both Russia and its highest peak. We wished each other well and then headed to our gates. Wardrobe can be so important, right? Keep paying attention to other people's T-shirts, I reminded myself. They can lead to making new friends.

By the time I reached Los Angeles International, I needed food and drink. Good old LAX: enchilada soup and a Budweiser beer rang up to $15. Then, I hustled to catch the shuttle bus to my Melbourne, Australia, gate connection. What was I thinking? I then sat for multiple hours awaiting departure. Once on board the plane I would sit multiple more hours, 15 plus to be precise. The time variance with Indiana is 16 hours, and Australia is ahead of the US. I believed I could keep this straight using 12 hour increments. This knowledge would help me avoid making three A.M. phone calls to friends and family.

A 22-year old Australian guy named Travis sat beside me on the plane. With a mate, Travis had spent the last six months traveling the USA and Canada. "To be so young and seeing the world—what a gift," I said to him.

Travis and I talked over our meal and a beverage. Sleep was in my immediate future, I hoped, but the aircraft temperature was exceedingly warm. Arrgh. And then our ride turned bumpy. Aarrgh again. On the plane's sound system I listened to Aussie Aboriginal music. Oh, I liked this: drums, chants, some kind of flute-like wind instrument . . . all of which provided peace to my own turbulence. Soon I fell asleep.

I awakened and visited with Travis again. His answers to my questions helped me formulate a plan. He knew the south-east of Australia where I would be. My entire trip was without a single overnight reservation. I didn't like doing it this way and usually firmed up the details of my trips in advance, but my 12 days Down Under would be fluid and fairly quick-paced.

When was the last time you left home not knowing where you'd spend the next night, let alone the next 12 nights? I certainly wasn't homeless and I don't wish to connect my circumstance with those so challenged. But my situation gave me some insight to the work of Wheeler Mission Ministries in Indy, which I modestly support. So I said prayers for Wheeler Mission's work to help the hungry, homeless, and unemployed.

I would travel through the territories of New South Wales and Victoria. In consultation with Travis, I outlined my sketchy plan of driving from Melbourne to Mount Kozzie, which was halfway to Sydney. Although Kozzie was my first objective and principally why I came to Australia, I did have additional objectives on this trip. Joe and Linda Heldt, longtime friends in Columbus who traveled to Australia, suggested I climb the Sydney Harbour Bridge.

"Why not?" I asked myself. After all, I'd be in the neighborhood. After Kozzie would come Sydney. Then my final objective involved heading west back to Melbourne, stopping somewhere halfway for an overnight or two. My return to Melbourne was to attend the Australian Open, which the Heldts also saw on their visit.

The Australian Open is a classic international tournament—one of the four Grand Slam world tennis attractions. As a tennis buff I was excited about this, although I didn't have a ticket. That would be another "i" to dot along the way.

I thanked Travis for his companionship and counsel. Though he hadn't trekked his homeland's Seven Summit peak of Kozzie, during the state-side expedition he and his mate climbed Half-Dome at Yosemite National Park. I had tried that the previous summer, two weeks after summiting Mount Elbrus in Russia. I was on Half Dome with Gretchen Scherschel Seibert and her husband Matt. Once I started going up Half Dome I realized how much of me I'd left in Russia. I needed to turn around below the "ladders," just beneath the Dome's summit.

Yet what a blast it was being with Gretchen and Matt. I have always told Gretch's parents, my good friends Greg and Peggy Scherschel, "If I had a daughter, it'd be Gretchen." Gretchen and Matt, a lovely and strong young couple, trekked 50 miles across the California mountains from Mammoth Ski Resort where they live and work to catch-up with me at Yosemite where I was vacationing with my college buddies and their spouses. What a blast it was being with them. Travis reminded me of this lovely strong young couple with his climb of Half Dome.

We parted company on landing and I complemented Travis on his knowledge of this vast land. The itinerary he suggested worked well for me—another kindness.

Tuesday, January 11, 2011

Somewhere on the flight, Monday had merged into Tuesday. After skipping over much of the Pacific Ocean, the skies, the terra firma, and the time zones were literally down under.

Customs went zoom-zoom quick, as did passport control, and the currency exchange—a young queen gracing the five dollar bills. Car rental also was expeditious. Ah...there it was—the steering wheel was indeed on the wrong side of the car. Welcome to the reverse wackiness and dizziness. I trembled through the next two weeks behind that steering wheel as I drove on what was, for me, the wrong side of the road.

The Brisbane couple in Indy had suggested a GPS—what a great idea—and this new friend's persistent female voice helped me clear the airport traffic and find the proper freeway. I grew a bit tired of hearing her say, "Recalculating," and her subsequent directives escalated from bossiness to sounding like threats. The female Australian voice I'd chosen began to get huffy with me. Do they program them that way, or was it my imagination? Heck, I even made the poor woman stutter.

After an hour of tedious interstate driving I moved onto a two lane highway. I was all about concentration behind the wheel, on the wrong side of the car, with the car on the wrong side of the road. If you've ever experienced driving in this manner, especially for the first time, you'll understand my mounting motoring angst, uncertainty, and disbelief. Ultimately, the driving became cautious fun. Still, I've never been honked at so much. And I got it: "It's me you're honking at, mates I know. It's me. My bad. My bad again. And again." Somehow I muddled through—angels must've taken pity on me.

In one town I circled the same roundabout four times, trying to exit at the correct spot. I totally exasperated the voice on the GPS box, who kept saying "Recalculating." I wondered if the rental car staff took bets on how quickly their American clients and other wrong-side rookies would crash the cars.

I soon saw firsthand the severe flooding in South Wales and neighboring territories. Rains had been extraordinarily heavy and the radio's updated news reports augmented the Brisbane couple's advisory. As I drove northeast toward Mount Kozzie and the Snowy Mountains, an hour's stretch of road looked ready for Noah and company to pull up anchor. Any more rain would imperil the road I drove on. In spots, a huge lake had overflowed its shoreline and the water lay only 50 to 100 feet from the highway. To me, the lake resembled the Tasman Sea or the South Pacific Ocean, but roadside signs said this was some big fresh water lake. Mental Note: Plan another return route back to Melbourne. This road might soon be ready for Noah's zoo.

On I drove, and made another discovery. As much as there was "water, water everywhere," as the poet Coleridge wrote, my car had less and less petrol in the tank. Uh, oh. A low gas gauge was a minor problem back home, even in rural Indiana, because small towns with gas stations dotted the countryside. Not so in Australia, where everything spread out—way out. The needle on my gauge was starting to bottom out and not a county seat or village was in sight. All I saw were what we'd call ranches out west in America. Coleridge also wrote of an important attribute in his poem "The Rhyme of the Ancient Mariner:" suspend disbelief. Accordingly, I said prayers, suspended disbelief, and drove virtually on empty for a long while, hoping and praying for a petrol stop. And when I surely was on my final fume, a petrol station in a three or four building town showed up. Thank you, God, and Samuel Taylor Coleridge.

Think of a convenience store in the USA. What do you see inside? Self-serve soda fountains, coffee bars, candy bars, popcorn, hot dogs, packaged food, and shelves with magazines and newspapers. My lovely oasis shelves offered fish bait, bullets, beer, ranch supplies, dry goods, saddles and tack, and camping material. It was a general all-purpose mercantile store appropriate for out in the middle of ranchland where it was situated. No USA mini-mart stuff in sight.

I went in to pay for the petrol in advance. You know, like we sometimes do in Indiana. I got a funny look straight-away when I pulled out my billfold.

"Mate, you haven't put any petrol in your tank yet. You have to put your petrol in your tank first. Right," the proprietor declared, looking at me like I was a teenager from Mars. "Otherwise, how do I know what you owe?"

Lamely I said something about how it worked at home.

He was having none of it. "Go put the petrol in your car man and then come pay me, right."

I wondered if my GPS Commander was the guy's sister. The proprietor wore a straw hat like one of our western ranch hands or cowboys. And he ruled this general store. He was friendly enough, and he happily confirmed where my paper map had told me about where I was. Soon enough his "sister" who ruled my driving would agree with what her brother said—I was getting close to the National Park named for its prominent feature, Mount Kosciuszko.

His parting words were like a benediction blessing. "Good idea you stopped mate. This here's your last drop of petrol 'til you get to the park town."

Oh, geez. Thank you, God, again. This was sheep country, as I'd seen them all about. I don't remember seeing any, crops, but neglected to ask about this, however. Sheep there are as important as corn crops in my county and state. Maybe you know Indiana produces more corn for popping than 49 other states, and in fact

20 per cent of the national supply of such. Looking about me and seeing all the grazing white fluff, I wondered if Australia made a similar claim for sheep production.

I was keen to see another kind of Aussie animal, a kangaroo, or 'Roo. None of those were to be seen hereabouts, nor were there any of the unusual other animals of Australian lore, like a koala or a wallabee. Thankfully, none of the deadly spiders I was wary of had put in an appearance either.

Back in my red car, I motored on—me and my kit and a full load of petrol zipping down the road's wrong side. Traffic was light; a good thing as my driving was still a work in progress. The terrain became washboard hills, still ranch country with few houses and fewer towns. The country was green from all the rain, yet it seemed arid. Something else about my driving—occasionally my wheelmanship let the left rear tire go off the roadway. Dang. I needed to be mindful of this and compensate for it.

I missed Lori. I missed Dom and family, Andy and family. I missed driving on my side of the road, and on my side of the car. I swear the GPS Commando said, "You are a whiner."

Does Kossie's real name sound familiar to you? The name Kosciuszko will sound familiar to some Hoosiers because in northern Indiana we have a county named after the same Polish war hero: Tadeusz Kosciuszko. Somehow a close friend of Thomas Jefferson, this revered Polish solider fought on the American side in the Revolutionary War. I know—you read it here first!

This was as far south of the equator as ever I'd been. The balmy temps of 70 felt good compared to Indiana winter. No wonder I felt tired—I'd been on the move for the past 50 to 60 hours, although I napped occasionally on the flights. GPS Commando: "You are whining again." My fatigue would soon be exacerbated by two episodes of angst, both financial: $16 and $149.

The $16 was what I owed the National Park to enter the park. However, I was unsuccessful in finding the location to pay this fee on the way in. So it went unpaid–not because I was a scofflaw, but because I saw no one to take my money. I felt like a trespasser, which bothered me. I didn't have an admission sticker and receipt to show anyone who wanted to see them. Unlike the U.S.A., where state and national parks have a little sentry post on the way in, this admissions ticket booth was off the road somewhere tucked within a village building. Despite asking, I was unable to find it. Arggh. I could almost see the headline: "American Clergy Held in Mountain Park Jail Over $16 Fee."

Well I needed to keep moving, so I drove up a long winding mountain road for half an hour. Having passed no park service or law enforcement vehicle, I drove into the national park village and located a hotel.

"Yes, we have one room available—a single. The price is $149. Would you like it?" I heard the hotel clerk say.

"Gulp," I heard me say. Had I paid $149 per night for an overnight stay, anywhere, I wondered? Noooo.

"Tell you what," I said to the clerk, "I just arrived. I'm going to go shopping first. Let me see what I turn up." He understood. "Will my vehicle be okay in your lot?"

"Yes sir."

I asked the kindly clerk to recommend other places and he did so.

I encountered crowds, and several small hotels I shopped could only offer one night's stay. "The Summer Jazz Festival Week is on mate," I was told. I learn the Festival is huge, and well-attended big deal, featuring names of fame. Great! I continued searching and found a nice lodge with a friendly manager who had a room for one night, at about half the hotel's rate. I snapped it up.

The downside: the Jazz Festival brought registered lodgers coming and would result in my premature eviction. But the owner urged me to stay, saying he would try to arrange something—"But no promises." I was on the one-day-at-a-time plan.

From Ed Viesturs, America's great mountain climber, I learned to compartmentalize. Compartmentalize? Yes. Let me explain. Compartmentalizing, Ed Viesturs taught me, means dealing with today's issues today, and not getting ahead of oneself. Viesturs is a hero for me—the first American to climb all the world's 8,000 meter peaks and he did it without the assistance of bottled oxygen. Can you imagine this undertaking? It too him 18 years to accomplish this feat. Patience please, Walter!

Imagine taking two decades to complete the climbs. Day in and day out over two decades, working to achieve a dream— astounding and awesome. So much for today's culture of instant gratification. When first accomplished, this was an unbelievable undertaking. Even today he is one of the few people to climb all the 8,000 meter mountains on Planet Earth. Fewer still have done so without oxygen.

I have an autographed copy of Viesturs' book courtesy of my friends at Rainier Mountaineering Inc. in Ashford, WA. My friends got his autograph for me after I fell on Rainier during my first time climbing with RMI. Because of my early exodus due to the fall, I wasn't able to meet Ed and personally ask him to sign the book. Having it arrive in the mail at my home was a nice consolation prize for not summiting Rainier.

"Compartmentalize. Focus on the issues before you," he says in the book. Physicians call this *triage* when they take care for the most critical patients first. In daily life it means doing the headline items on my calendar first when I have enthusiasm and energy borne of sunrise, before I grow weary of doing the B and C secondary tasks.

Mind you, all are important or they wouldn't be on my calendar. And when people came to my open office door, it was right to abandon the calendar and see to their immediate needs.

As I see it, compartmentalizing is the wisdom of knowing what to do first—and to be flexible and resilient while following the process so you can commit with strength to action. Jesus calls this, "separating the wheat from the chaff." I cobbled this into Psalm 37's verses 1, 3, and 5, and tell myself: "Do not worry. Beget calmness and poise for me on the mountain, in my hospital ministries, and my personal life."

So, here in Australia, I accepted the lodging situation without getting ahead of myself. The lodge manager Ted signed me up for one night and promised to look into a second night. Good to go.

I checked the St. Vincent Blackberry to look for posts on my newly created blog 2trek4kids.org. There I found a lovely note from Lori. In fact, I found a number of posts, all greatly appreciated. Thanks to Scott Cox, Ph.D. at St. Vincent Salem Hospital for creating the blog from scratch.

Thredbo, the town here in the Kosciuszko National Park, is a ski resort town. I found a restaurant for dinner and looked out on the base of a ski lift across the creek below. I also noticed a familiar scent later as I walked through the village—warm wax that would be applied to skis before summer storage. I also smelled the rain that had begun falling. Even though summer had arrived Down Under, I saw the lift running, though obscured by rain clouds as it went upward. The elevation gain was a mere 560 feet—not much compared to the mountains I ski in Colorado, but I wished it were winter so I might ski Australia as well as trek there. I reminded myself that skiing Down Under would mean I wasn't there for the world class Grand Slam Tennis event.

Awaiting dinner, I journaled and thought about being a world away from home, this time by myself. I had no expedition crew, guides, or fellow trekkers to befriend me, which is something all the other mountains provided me as gift. The scent of a pork sausage something or other dish took my mind off the journal.

Seeing the incongruence of Thredbo's ski lift rising through lush green growth instead of white snow, I remembered the Mount Elbrus trip with Lori six months earlier and watching Russians ski during the northern hemisphere's summer on Elbrus' permanent snowfield. Here I was in the southern hemisphere again—as with Africa where Kili is three degrees south of the equator. And here before me was another of the world's Seven Summits. How blessed I felt, though still a bit lonely. I decided I should get used to talking to myself and responding to the GPS female commando in my car.

Thursday, January 13, 2011

I slept like a little boy and awakened to delightful birdsong and sunlight. A warm shower felt great and dissipated yesterday's "fragrance." I checked the Blackberry and found more posts to the blog, including from son Andy and from Sherrie Schmidt, pediatric nurse practitioner at St. Vincent Salem who cared for many of the children in the youth obesity program. Also messages from more family, colleagues, and children of colleagues. I might have been alone, but I was not by myself. And in mountain environments I especially feel God's presence.

For person-to-person interaction I ran into Ted, the proprietor of Bernti's where I was staying. A nice man, he provided information about the Kozzie trek and breakfast options. I followed his recommendation to a nice, nearby outdoor café. I like me coffee black and bold, and ordered accordingly. I am a four cup java man at breakfast (and rare it is for me to drink java after breakfast), but two "Long Blacks" at this cafe turned the coffee trick. I devoured a fair-sized breakfast of scrambled eggs and toast, and then settled on the idea of going for the summit that day. Ted said there was the likelihood of rain the on this day, but tomorrow would be even wetter. I brought rain gear, but wanted to enjoy a dry uphill walk, if possible.

Reaching this decision, I finished breakfast in gulps and bites. Growing eager, I returned to Bernti's and prepared purposefully and in haste. I originally thought this would be an acclimatization day, but the plan had changed and I needed to take care of business. God willing, Seven Summits # 4 was coming up.

As I packed my backpack and dressed, I thought of two things: a) My other summit day preparations at Mount Everest Base Camp, Mount Kilimanjaro, and Mount Elbrus. Each of those required rising early and investing long days; and, b) Those to whom the climbs were dedicated: The children and families of the L.I.F.E (Lifetime Individual Fitness and Eating) for Kids clinical programs in southern Indiana and St. Vincent hospitals. I also thought of the dedicated, compassionate, and competent clinicians, like Lori and high-energy Jackie Kramer.

I laced up my boots and then slid on my pack. This mountain of 7,310 feet did not require the extensive summit day preparations of previous peaks. But I would remain humble lest one of those poisonous Aussie spiders of Kozzie bite me. Now was the time to empower the dedications. Out the door I went.

When I walked across the street and onto the creek bridge over the creek, people were already boarding the ski lift to gain the 500 foot front end mountain access. I joined them, thinking how nice these ski lifts were for mountain hiking or—like me—going for the summit. The temperature was 59 degrees, wind freshening, light to moderate, and no rain so far. A short lift ride of a few minutes deposited us at the trailhead and I headed for the lowest of the Seven Summits—but still one of the fabled Seven.

I left the hotel at 10:46 a.m. and returned at 3:46 p.m. Five hours, and it was done! I reached the top of the 7,310 foot summit and came back down the ski lift. My Virgin Health Miles Go Zone pedometer said I trekked 8.2 miles, which seemed a little short given that it also told me I recorded 18,642 steps. It said my caloric burn was 724. The weather was mild, but included spotty drenching rain. This delightfully reminded me of our Everest descent day to Namchee Bazaar when it rained for hours at a time. The rain stopped when I summited today, but clouds hid the view. On my descent, the rain resumed and ended in a downpour that left me soaked.

Rather than a traditional rendering of the day's events, because Kozzie was so different, I will share impressions from my journal based on the five senses.

-Sounds

The melody of small waterfalls gurgling downward as I passed by—some coming from lingering snowfields still visible in the distance, though it was summer time. The snowfields I saw in the distance were sheltered from the sun.

The brittle call of one of Kozzie's many crows, this one particularly close by. The bird looked my way and seemed to be fussing at me. I asked aloud the crow and his neighbors, "Are you Down Under cousins to the crows Lori and I saw at Elbrus in Russia? Or are you kin to the Goraks (crows) at Gorak Shep (at Everest loosely translated from the Nepalese as Crow's Nest), the last human outpost four hours down from Everest Base Camp?" The Kozzie crow turned its head, stared at me and, cawed again. I had no translation for what it said. Probably my imagination, but at the end I thought I heard it caw "mate."

Tinkling rainfall, gentle at first, and then a pummeling tom-tom hard on my plastic outerwear. This was not a commercially made poncho. Last worn at the Louisville Mini Marathon the previous May, it was a 50 gallon heavy duty plastic contractor's bag I modified for poncho purposes. This light weight raingear was perfect for the day. Maybe it was my imagination, but the raindrops sounded different in gentleness and force as they splashed on the garbage bag rather than onto a true manufactured poncho.

The sound of the gentle wind's movement, almost like the Hebrew word "ruah" or Greek "pneuma" for "wind" or "spirit."

The squeaky press of my boot soles on the iron grated walkway that rose a foot or two above the tundra. The walkway ensured we didn't destroy the beautiful wildflowers along the track. The walkway was a simple, yet remarkable, feat of engineering and profound wisdom. It turned and twisted up the mountainside. Kozzie is a gentle, rising slope, not steep like the other six summits. The three foot wide grated walkway protected the environment and was present for about half of the trail. I carried and used my trek poles for much of the route. Their utility on the grate was useless, and in fact the carbide tips got caught between the rods when first I tried them. They proved totally ineffective on the metal grate and made a striking metallic noise. Carbide tip on metal grate was a clanging cymbal compared to the muted, soft sound of my boot treads as the soles squeaked on moisture between the sole and the grate. After the trek poles got tangled inside the grate spaces, they went silent as I shouldered them.

The voices of other trekkers were among my favorite sounds.

"Guh day, Mate!"

"How are you going along?"

"How you going today?"

English spoken by Australians sounded cheerful and lively. I also enjoyed children's voices, especially two youngsters I followed. There was the enthusiasm, and weariness, of two young girls hiking up with their parents. I'd say they were four or five years old. I met up with them near the top and I complimented the wee ones on how well they were doing. Shy, they smiled wanly and looked more at their mom and dad than me. The dad, using adult language, allowed the younger was struggling. Yet both little girls soldiered on. The children talked to their folks as I walked along with the family for a bit. I like how children sound, and with their nuanced Aussie speak these girls were a delight to listen to. Their questions were the ageless ones of children, spoken from tiredness. I heard: "When will we be there?" I stifled a laugh. The girls were dressed alike in mostly white. As a dad who has laundered kid's clothes I thought, "Hmmm, wonder how white that will look at the end of this wet and muddy day?" I hung with them for a bit, happy for the company and delighted to be in the presence of children. Finally, I bid them a "good day" and pressed on, resuming my pace. We met again later—at the top when the family summited, all of them together. I went right up to each girl and exclaimed: "Congratulations. You are on top of one of the Seven Summits of the World! I expect you're the youngest people today to stand on top! Bravo! Well Done!" And in my best Aussie I used a local expression, "Good on you." I hope that made it more special for the girls. I know the parents beamed.

I took pics with my Blackberry camera and Lori's camera I borrowed. The fourth of the Seven Summits—I needed pics for the blog and for archives—also for Siena, and hopefully other grandkids in the wings and wombs.

I head miscellaneous sounds:

Snapping my backpack open and closed...a slight breeze that continually caressed the wildflowers...more crows...and as the rain resumed I heard it again on my plastic skin. Finally, I listened to my own breath move easily in and out—no need here for the pressure breathing used at high elevations to help oxygenate the lungs to move air efficiently.

-Touch

I collected 43 small rocks for gifts and felt their wetness, dirt, and sediment on my fingers. My feet inside my boots felt strong and limber. My legs were also strong and limber. I felt the unnatural lightness of the pack I carried, its only weight coming from three liters of water and the rocks I collected. I noticed the feel of Andy and Jill's Christmas gift—a gray Columbia fleece jacket, and also the snack bar I unwrapped, the cork grips of the trek poles, and the gentle breeze caressing my face. My plastic garbage bag covering and the clothes just underneath were damp on the outside from rain, and on the inside from perspiration.

-Smells

I noted the scent of the hand sanitizer I used before snacking, drinking, or using the camera. I smelled the Gatorade original lemon-lime powder product mix. Later in the day, I smelled a Kosciuszko Brewing Company Pale Ale when I celebrated this fourth of the Seven Summits to climb on, and third of four to summit. And, finally:

-Sights

From the track I could see the snowfields far away and green plants beside and below the walkway. Purple and pink daisy-like flowers grew everywhere, even near the snow. The rock formations, the tallest maybe 40 feet high, were stark and rough in appearance, resembling the outside of a geode. I admired the metal grate for its conception, engineering design, and construction, which included contoured cuttings around boulders. The grate rose and fell, blending man's talent with God's terrain.

As the rain fell, more clouds moved in and then slowly dissipated to give me a brief, snapshot view of the valley below. A monument near the summit marked this as the highest point on the continent of Australia. Nearby stood a large triangulation rock structure constructed for measuring elevation—before we had GPS. Heading downward, I enjoyed catching a ride on the ski lift, moving above the January greenery Down Under, and returning to my starting point.

Back at the hotel, feeling gleeful about the summit ascent, I was cleared for another night at Bernti's place. Thank you, God, and Ted, and also the drummer of the jazz band who would spend the night with one of his mates instead of his (my) room.

Friday, January 14, 2011

I begin my day naming names for God using Scriptural references and ran the tally up near 200. More than an academic exercise, this daily practice had become a kind of prayer for giving glory to God.

Time for some java and sustenance, or "breaky" as they call it in Australia. I learned the word from the British culture at Everest, where its use was prevalent. Brits were among the first pioneers and most famous of mountain climbers, so their culture influences climbing locales around the world. And of course English culture remains prevalent in Australia—their former colony.

Before turning in the night before, I forwarded a brief summit account to the blog. By morning, congratulations came in from all, including Lori.

Speaking of Lori, I finally heard her voice again after numerous attempts to connect. I brought her up to date on my time Down Under. Regarding the quick summit of Kozzie, Lori referenced our Russia climb and its many ordeals. Then she deadpanned one of my mountaineering career's classic action lines:

"That Australian mountain was so easy. Heck, you should do it again!"

I laughed and reply, "I'd considered that, but it's supposed to pour rain today. I got wet enough yesterday. I don't need that again. My things are just starting to dry out from rain and then my hand washing to get 'em clean."

I told Lori what was percolating inside my head: "Okay, the mountain is done and I've been given one more night here. The proprietor was great making accommodations for me. He persuaded members of the jazz band staying next door, who also had this room, to let me use it tonight. So I plan to check out early tomorrow morning and head for Sydney so I can climb the Sydney Harbour Bridge. I'll stay there a bit, and then start making my way back to Melbourne for the Australian Open. And before we know it I'll be back home again in Indiana. I can hardly wait to see you! "

With the plan made and spoken, I figured out my morning. Breaky and gift shopping were accomplished in short order, so I took a stroll around the village. I followed the creek, starting near the ski lift in the mercantile area of the village, where I smell ski wax again. The mountain village of Thredbo is an attractive area, befitting a national park. Its rustic appeal reminded me of Nashville, next door to me in Brown County, Indiana. The streets were clean and friendly, with people speaking to each other in Aussie accents. Following the creek, I admired condos built into the hillside, the building materials, colors, and condo lines blending nicely with the environment.

Up ahead, a bend in the road paralleled a bend in the creek. Nestled in a woodsy area, I saw a glass-walled building facing the creek and forest beyond. Then I noticed a low steeple with a cross on top. Perfect! A Christian sacred space in a beautiful natural setting. Upon walking closer, I was struck by the impressive building that, at first, seemed disarmingly small and simple. It turned out to be a Catholic Church and gathering space called the John Paul II Catholic Center. Admiring its elements, I thought, "I'd like to meet the architect and have him give me a walkabout." The back side of the church facing the woods was entirely glass. From the outside looking in, I saw the architect had situated the altar on that end, so the worshipping congregation would look out toward the green space of God's woods, with the priest facing his congregation. All streets, parking, houses, poles, or wires were precluded from the view. This was an impressive use of natural beauty.

I appreciate innovative sacred spaces like this church—and I don't necessarily mean big cathedrals or basilicas. Small churches like this one bring art and architecture to small communities where congregations may never have the opportunity to worship in a huge gathering space like a cathedral or basilicas located in populated areas. The Old Testament goes into fair detail in 1 Kings: Chapters 5 and 6, about the building of temples and the use of stone. The author of 1 Peter: Chapter 2 seems to pick up on this by calling Jesus the "living stone," and saying people also are like "living stones being built into a spiritual house."

I was involved in the chapel design for three different St. Vincent Hospital ministries: St. Vincent Jennings, Salem, and Dunn. These projects blessed me with a unique opportunity to collaborate in the design of contemporary worship spaces that convey sacred expression. This work united me with creative architects, planners, artisans, and our associates—all with good ideas. These experiences gave me, so to speak, a new set of eyes.

My first chapel project was for St. Vincent Jennings in North Vernon, where a new building project included a totally new sacred space for the hospital ministry. A few years before I had a budding interest in stained glass windows and visited several Catholic and non-Catholic churches to pursue this. I wasn't a passive visitor. Thanks to former neighbor and friend Nolan Bingham, himself an architect, I read a professional publication devoted to articles and photographs on American churches, mosques, and synagogues. At one time I think I was the only non-architect with a subscription to the American Association of Architects "Faith and Forum" magazine. Through reading the magazine, and seeing real-life views of sacred spaces at home and in my travels, I was becoming a casual student.

When I was missioned to Jennings I learned about their new construction project costing $14 million to upgrade the entire facility. Rosemary Hume, my St. Vincent mentor, spoke to me of the new chapel and said that, as chaplain, I would be the point person for its construction. I was delighted at this opportunity to cobble my private interest in sacred worship spaces with my professional calling.

For the last several years, during my travels I often visited churches to see what the designers were up to. I visited a number of Indy area churches too, including a Jewish Temple, where my friend Rabbi Arnold even asked me to present to his congregation on the eve of the High Holy Days—one of my life's highest spiritual honors. I so appreciated my tour of the synagogue and its heritage, art, and architecture.

Catholic identity is essential to St. Vincent chapels, including plans for new chapels. Perhaps from the rejections elsewhere when I was unable to see the inside of a church, I knew I wanted our chapels to provide spiritual hospitality to other Christian religions, welcoming un-churched patients and families, along with people from other faith traditions.

I collaborated with William Fenton, St. Vincent's facilities architect. We also involved William "Buzz" Weberding from Weberding Carving Shop in Batesville, IN, near Cincinnati. Buzz, whose name was also Bill, joined St. Vincent's Bill on most all of the St. Vincent Hospital chapel designs. On the southern Indiana St. Vincent projects, I joined the team. Bill and Buzz were exceptional to work with.

I also collaborated on a St. Vincent chapel in Indianapolis, at the St. Vincent Heart Center. I would see more of that chapel as an open heart surgery patient after my fall on Mount Rainier in 2012. Chapels, in my language, are the spiritual centerpieces of our hospitals, I'd tell people. "First we shape our buildings, and then our buildings shape us," a quote from Winston Churchill.

Part of our healing ministry, St. Vincent Hospital chapels have been included in our hospitals for the 130 and more years we've been in Indianapolis and Hoosier communities. I wanted to build on our heritage and hoped the result would make all our hospital ministry constituents feel welcome. With my Columbus roots and its remarkable connection to architecture and my interest in sacred spaces, perhaps I could provide architectural amenities to make them special.

With help from Bill and Buzz, we created small spaces of simple elegance in which through Buzz' cherry liturgical furniture, Bill's footprint, and the most beautiful of stained glass windows, which I helped coordinate, we honored God and welcomed visitors. I wanted the chapels to be welcoming for our hospital patients and families, associates, physicians, and guild members—plus people in our communities. I hope and believe the chapels glorify God and uplift people through the spaces themselves and the services conducted there.

Borrowing and adapting a story from the building of one of Columbus' most beautiful churches, I teased Buzz about each new chapel we created. I painted for Buzz a vision of his appearance at the gate of Heaven. I told him: "When you get in front of St. Peter at the Pearly Gates, he's gonna say: 'Hello Buzz, and welcome. I have a question for you. What work among all of your most beautiful sacred spaces do you find the most beautiful?'"

And then I told, "Buzz, you should be prepared to say . . ." When we were in North Vernon working on the Jennings Chapel I told him to identify the Jennings chapel to St. Peter. Then came Salem and he was told to note the Salem Chapel; and, then at Bedford he was instructed to identify that chapel. Each of these chapels is beautifully distinctive in its own way.

There was even a fourth chapel, albeit only for a day. When it came time to bless and dedicate the chapel at St. Vincent Dunn, in Bedford, my hometown, I invited our new Archbishop Joseph Tobin, fresh to Indianapolis from duties at the Vatican, to celebrate the Mass. He has since been elevated to Cardinal Joseph. The Indianapolis Archdiocese's 38 south-central Indiana counties, for which he was shepherd, included Lawrence county, where St. Vincent Dunn was located. When Cardinal Joseph graciously accepted my invite, holy smokes, there was no way the beautiful new 14 seat chapel would accommodate the throng of worshippers we expected. So with the help of a cast of thousands at Dunn (or so it seemed) we converted the hospital's large fitness center into a chapel for day. And 100 people filled it up for the most beautiful of Masses, courtesy of Cardinal Joseph.

So when I saw the Aussie national park's village of Thredbo had such a beautiful Catholic church and center named for a pope who is now canonized as a saint, I wanted to go inside. Sadly, the building was locked. In a couple of days I'd worship within a historic church for royals at the foot of the Sydney Harbour Bridge, plus I would visit a historical sacred space in Melbourne.

As I returned to the lodge, gray clouds that were hanging overhead all morning unleashed the predicted heavy downpour. Soon, the rain turned into a deluge. "If this is the weather we have in the valley, what's it like on the mountain top?" I asked myself. Thankfully, I'd already reached the summit and now I could stay dry.

From my window I saw people in the street, soaked from head to toe and wearing dripping backpacks. They had probably just returned from the mountain. I hung out in my dry, cozy room and watched a movie on the tube. At dinner I visited with a guy who offered advice on where to stay in Sydney. My fellow diner published a ski magazine and owned a shop in the village.

Saturday, January 15, 2011

This was the travel day to Sydney, which took 6.5 hours, a little longer than I was told—probably because I had to drive over the Sydney Harbour Bridge twice. With the help of my GPS advisor, I successfully reached my destination.

I enjoyed the drive from the mountain to Sydney, with many warning signs to be on the watch for kangaroos. Too bad for me, I didn't see a one—or koalas, or wallabees. Driving into Sydney I heard a lawnmower and smiled to myself, remembering it was January and back home we'd be using noisy snow blowers. Plus, my eyes got a jolt as I spied surfboards atop many cars. Not something you see at all in Indiana. I got into the spirit of the Sydney summer and sunburned my right arm where it rested on the car's window ledge.

I drove without a mistake, thanks to my GPS guide with whom I was in perfect harmony at last, and we successfully reached the district where I intended to find lodging. Not a single hotel was in sight. I checked with the district locals who advised me to return downtown. This meant I had to drive back across the Sydney Harbour Bridge.

The bridge is perfectly massive—hundreds of feet above the water, hundreds of feet tall, and about eight lanes wide. A mass of steel girders, the bridge looked as if a giant's child had gone playful with his erector set. While driving across I had vertigo issues, especially when I was in motion, from driving the car so high up. The vertigo had happened to me before up high on bridges. It was probably exacerbated by the fact that this was the bridge I planned to climb.

While driving on the bridge I kept my bearings, pretty much, by focusing straight ahead. On the return trip across I peeked up at the bridge span where the climb went and troubles developed. Vertigo seized me, causing my hands to go clammy on the steering wheel. I involuntarily gripped the wheel even tighter. My tummy, which had felt fine, went into knots. I found myself involuntarily slowing the car. The solution was to look absolutely straight ahead. On the bridge, on this occasion, I had to mentally block out the idea of climbing this sucker. My symptoms continued as I drove into the heart of downtown Sydney, one of the world's largest cities, to find a hotel—in an area I hoped was near the bridge.

Having said a prayer for convenient parking, I found a perfect place to park right across from the Vibe Hotel in Sydney. And believe it or not, the place had an available room. But holy moley—the rooms cost $225 a night—way over my budget.

I was numb from driving, especially the pair of bridge crossings, so I didn't want to get back into my car and drive around looking for another hotel. I swallowed hard and took the room after thanking God for an inn and a room at the inn, exorbitant as the cost was. Then some fairly good news developed. It turned out a second night only cost $110. This averaged out to $162 a night—more than the national park hotel price at which I had so blanched only a few days ago, but better than I first thought. Plus, the foot of the Sydney Harbour Bridge was only a few blocks away. Had that parking space not opened up, this chapter might have taken a different turn. I once heard there are parking lot angels we can pray to—but that was a joke, right?

My room was an ordinary twin bed offering, with no television. I didn't mind not having the TV set, but found this unbelieveable at the price. At least the off-street locked garage parking was free, the desk clerk said. "Lucky me," I deadpanned. Ah, but when I needed the parking space saint—she had delivered.

I missed Lori. I missed Siena and Dom and Kathryn. I missed Andy and Jill. Heck, I even missed the voice of my GPS female compass with whom I'd established a sort-of relationship.

Sunday, January 16, 2011

At 30 minutes after midnight, Lori called on my Blackberry. Lunchtime at home. I emerged from a deep sleep, always glad to hear from her. She spoke of home, daughters, and youth obesity prevention and treatment matters. I recounted getting to Sydney and seeing the gigantic Harbour Bridge up close and personal—twice.

"It's one of the biggest, if not the biggest, bridge in the world. It carries vehicles, locomotive traffic, pedestrians, and bicycles. Not to mention climbers. It's high above the harbor and also quite tall. I was so taken by it I drove across twice!"

Lori sounded wide awake, bright, and cheery. I tried to equal her mood. She told me to do well and look good on the bridge climb, now only a few hours away.

The next morning was a Sunday, and I like to do some "extra credit" reading for scripture in Psalms. This morning I did a lectio divina reading of Chapter 46:10, the verse I wore on my backpack for all mountain expeditions: "Be still and know that I am God."

Lectio divina is the practice of choosing a verse or a few verses to reflectively read over and over again. Questions for me to explore that morning included: What was going on in the writer's life at the time he wrote the verse? What did this verse mean in the era in which it was written? Did it have application today, for me and for others? And what might that application be? What did God want me to get out of this reading?

I believe Psalm 46:10 refers to the importance of meditation, particularly meditating on nature in my life, and on God who made nature, or caused it to be made. It means taking time to develop an appreciative and grateful outlook about what God has given us in nature, including our bodies, minds, and spirits. I think too it refers not so much to physical stillness, but the quietness and peace of my inner spirit. And, I know that when I get quiet, or still, God may begin to reveal Himself to me. The busyness of everyday life and incessant sound can steal our peace and our connection to the Divine, I think.

I believe the psalmist writer who crafted these few words must have had a peaceful spirit, full of poise; a man who appreciated solitude and quiet. On the day he wrote these words, perhaps he was exposed to deafening noise and chaos in a busy marketplace and it drove him bananas. Thus he retreated to the stillness of a wooded hill or mountaintop and its natural serenity to find God after the turmoil stole his peace.

I also spend some time with Isaiah 52:7: "How beautiful upon the mountains are the feet of him who brings good news." Because this day would bring the Sydney Harbour Bridge climb, I substituted those words for "mountain" to make the words come alive for me.

And I read Philippians 4:13: "I can do all things through Jesus Christ who gives me strength." This last one reflects the boldness and humility of its author, the Apostle Paul.

Leaving the hotel, I bought a creamy croissant at a bakery and then headed toward the bridge to find the office selling bridge climbing tickets. The bridge wasn't hard to find—it stuck out above everything. I soon received yet another spiritual gift. On a street located beneath the bridge's floor, at the foot of a massive support structure, stood a tiny church.

My first thought was, "How cool! I can do a fly-by." That's a spiritual technique I learned from my aunt and Godmother, Angie Meno. On her way to a hot golf or tennis game, Angie would first drive past St. Vincent de Paul Church, in her town of Bedford, Indiana. Her purpose was simply to say, "Hi, God." This was an in-motion way to pay respect and homage. Having learned this from her, I still practice it today.

Well, the surprise was on me, because it was Sunday, the small church before me was an Anglican Church, and their service had just begun. The Anglican liturgy follows the Catholic Church's liturgy, from which it evolved and the little Sydney Anglican church I stepped into had an absolutely beautiful service. The $20 fee I didn't pay to the Kozzie National Park went into the collection plate, along with a prayer.

Afterward I stayed for what some stateside churches call coffee and donuts, except this was "tea and cakes." Hearing my accent, everyone wanted to know my story, and I obliged. They seemed impressed by the fact I travelled alone and had such an ambitious plan. They were keen on my desire to climb the bridge in their back yard—the harbor. The giant structure loomed over the ant-like church like a spidery super-structure of horizontal and vertical thick iron. The bridge was nicknamed the "coathanger" and "iron monstrosity."

The minister asked if I knew their church held significance for English royalty. I didn't, I said. It was nick named The Queen's Chapel, he told me, and added, "This is the sacred space where the English queen and the royals come to worship when they visit Sydney. On your way out, go back in and see Her Majesty's crown carved into the back wall."

I did so—and there it was on the pale yellow wall. This turned out to be a royal spiritual occasion for me, and a great way to begin my bridge adventure. Alas, Her Majesty the Queen wasn't present to meet me.

Near the church, I found a stairway and a bicycle access lane to the bridge, so up I went. The bridge climb has been going on since 1998 and is a sanctioned activity for which safety is the gold standard. In fact, the activity is so popular that reservations are encouraged. Prospective climbers fill out a ream of paperwork, provide additional personal answers to staff when deemed appropriate, and submit to a breathalyzer test. Bridge climbers switch out of their street clothes to wear climbing clothes and safety gear.

But is anything cheap in Sydney? The bridge climb was $208, more than a day lift ticket to ski in Colorado. I felt tension between my frugal inner self and my desire to go for it, no matter the cost. The price seemed as steep as some of the stairs and ladders on the climb.

The first thing I learned was humbling—I had arrived on the wrong side of the bridge. I would need to walk eleven football field lengths across the pedestrian passageway in order to reach the registration office, pay my admission, and go through the screening.

First, however I had to walk across. Looking down to the water level from a few hundred feet made me go clammy and I hadn't even signed up for the climb yet. Looking down a couple of times cured me of that curiosity. Thereafter I stayed on the inside of the pedestrian walkway, away from the side of the bridge. The bridge was about 10 people wide and wasn't crowded on a Sunday morning. I saw a couple of bicycles go by and couples pushing baby strollers.

My willies subsided on reaching the bridge office, on land, in a building by the bridge. I went inside to pay, register, be evaluated, change clothes, and hear the safety briefing.

The single top-bottom bridge garment we climbers wore included a built-in harness to which a safety cable was attached. One of the bridge crew fastened the cable securely into a rail mechanism that only crew could release. As we climbed, the cable tethered us to the bridge. The cable slid along within a waist-high railing mechanism the entire length of the climb. This effectively prevented a fall (or a suicidal leap) from the bridge.

We made our way outside the building onto a ready platform above the deck, or road level of the bridge. My earlier clamminess returned as we went up steps that took us about 20 feet above and to the side of the vehicular traffic. A two foot wide walking track led through what seemed to be the bowels of the bridge. We would make our way across this lower level of the bridge before starting our climb up.

I tried not to look at the automobile and truck traffic below. Not looking helped a lot—until a locomotive and train rumbled along on its track under the road deck, creating what felt like earthquake vibrations. I found myself clutching the railing, my clamminess intensifying. Quickly, I began three practices to help myself:

1. I looked at my feet, not straight ahead or outward toward the view, and certainly not upward.

2. I prayed.

3. I began conscious breathing—in through the nose—exhaling from the mouth.

As I had taught Lori in Russia, I was surrendering to the unknown, and basically learning it all over again. As I continued practicing my self-care re-directions, a measure of poise returned to me and the angst began to subside. On my out breaths I exhaled the toxic fear and anxiety. With each inhalation, I imagined breathing in the Holy Spirit. I breathed peace in, and exhaled angst and fret—and did so with intention. I continued to watch my feet and did not let my vision wander. The mass of steel surrounding us, combined with the cloudy weather, made the area inside the bridge dark. After about 15 minutes of walking we reached the point where we'd begin the climb up in earnest.

Holy shit. (Excuse French.)

Our climb would take us up one of the outside arches of the bridge!

This wasn't apparent right away because we used stairways and ladders to gain some height inside the bridge's bowels. I almost fainted when we came out from the inside of the bridge work and began going up along the arch.

One mercy of the body and the psyche is that we tend to remember the hurt, but we block out the specific intensity of the pain. Maybe I lapsed into unconsciousness or my initial bridge fears deleted my memory, but I just can't remember much about that first part of the bridge climb up the outside truss.

I was scared, I admit it. But I managed to regain some poise. I reminded myself I was a mountain climber and reviewed memories of previous climbs in tight spots. I began regaining my confidence.

This reminded me of a spiritual principle: When one surrenders to the unknown, fear and awe may shake hands. I had helped Lori understand this principle when she had her crisis of confidence climbing in Russia, but I needed to re-learn it on the bridge. In Lori's case, she was superbly fit to accomplish the Mt. Elbrus climb, but her mental and emotional doubts caused uncertainty and angst about the challenge.

The bridge in Sydney differed from mountain heights. I'd been on four of the Seven Summits, to the tops of three, and to Everest Base Camp. But this bridge exposed me to a different kind of height. This man-made giant bridge was one of the tallest in the world, 440 feet from the water level to the top arch of the bridge, with the Sydney skyline at eye level. I mean, we could practically see into the building windows. Even though we were cabled into the bridge, rendering a fall impossible, my vertigo kicked into overdrive and jump-started my angst.

The result was a vice grip that left me clinging to railings, cables, ladders, stairwell bannisters—anything my hands contacted. My tennis elbow went sore for all the literal hanging on I did. My palms were soaked with nervy sweat. I told myself often what I had heard the Aussies say, "No worries, mate."

Sometimes I looked up from my feet—curiosity arrived as my confidence returned. The major problem was seeing things in minute detail: Boats and cars in motion, itty bitty pedestrians, skyscraper tops at eye level, other climbers elsewhere on the bridge. Oh, my. We were on the edge—literally, as our pathway continued up and up the side support spire-like truss. It wasn't terribly steep—like climbing a forever upward stairway.

Gradually, I gained the ability to look around and take in the sights. By doing so, I was adjusting to the height; "acclimatizing" in mountain language. As we reached the summit of the bridge, remarkably, I found my tight grip began to relax. I looked around, even focusing on detail below. Another change: I began to visit more with the companions in my small climbing group.

Cabled into the bridge ahead of me was a grandmother from Sydney climbing the bridge for the second time. Today she'd brought long her husband and their two grandchildren. Behind me were three people who had been university classmates in upstate New York. One of them, Jill, was an ovarian cancer survivor who was a Steelers fan. Pittsburgh was in a National Football League playoff game on that day—and at that very moment, in fact. "Sorry mate. No radios, I-Pods or cameras allowed on the bridge," she was told by bridge climb staff. So she was experiencing Steeler-anxiety. When I mentioned that Lori ran the then youth obesity prevention and treatment program at the Peyton Manning Children's Hospital, Jill latched right onto the vague connection and started calling me "Peyton" for the Manning who then quarter-backed the NFL Indianapolis Colts.

Then we found another connection. Another of the three classmates had done contract work in Melbourne for the multi-national diesel engine builder Cummins Engine which has world headquarters in my home town. I visited with that classmate at one of the stops on the bridge where we saw the sights and heard bridge lore from Owen (first name) our lead guide. I spoke of one of my neighbors at home who was on short-term assignment for Cummins in Melbourne, but Jill's classmate didn't know Josh.

Organized stops along the route included one at the top span of the bridge—440 feet above water level. There a moment of grace occurred. My surrender caused fear to give way to awe at my surroundings. I continued visiting with my bridge mates and continued looking outward.

Owen, our guide, was an affable fellow who told the story of how an orange figured into the architectural design of the iconic Sydney Opera House, which we could see below us. To show a committee the design he had in mind, the opera house designer sectioned an orange and inverted the pieces as he reassembled them before the group. Jorn Utzon, a young and relatively unknown Danish architect, won a design competition to create this masterpiece of modern architecture. The bridge was completed in 1932 and took eight years to build with 14,000 people continuously employed in the building. At the time, they were among the highest paid people in Sydney.

On the way down, to my surprise, I mostly stopped holding onto the rails and trusted my feet to get me safely where I needed to go. I looked intently at the boats and ships. I purposefully gazed at the tops of the skyscrapers on a level with us. I didn't even panic when Owen spoke of sharks in the water below. I examined nests the seabirds made in the bridge scaffolding. God's winged creatures nearly 500 feet above the water were making themselves at home within the trusses of man's creation. Owen spoke of 16 people who died during construction of the bridge. He then added that, likewise, sometimes baby birds fell to their deaths from their steel and straw nests before learning to fly.

Feeling vibrations from a train rumbling underneath us, I smiled. No more death grip on the bridge railing. I was surrendering to the unknown. Fear and awe were shaking hands, which was so much better than my hands shaking in fear.

The trek and climb on the bridge was 4.5 hours without a bathroom break. My Go Zone pedometer from Virgin Health Miles measured the distance at approximately 2,000 steps, meaning we traveled up and down and across one mile.

On my walk back across the bridge to the side where my pricey hotel was located, I felt different than a few hours earlier. I walked the pedestrian access way with ease. No more willies or angst. The bridge climb was a confidence builder for me.

Gazing at the top of the bridge from below, I was a little in awe when I realized what I'd done and watched the next group make their climb. I documented my adventure by shooting Blackberry pictures from the bridge floor. And I laughed at the irony of having crossed the bridge multiple times in one day. I definitely set a new PR for bridge crossings in a day, exceeding the earlier number set in a car.

On my way to the Vibe I stopped at the first grocery after getting off the bridge and had a pastry. An array of colorful fresh fruit was displayed in baskets and boxes in front of the store right in the heart of the downtown. I went in to buy a banana, which I actually ate before paying. Hey, I was hungry and my blood sugar felt like it had bottomed out. The grocer looked a little dumbfounded when I shamefacedly gave him my peel and said, "Sorry! It was a big one, so charge me accordingly." We both laughed.

I decided fish and chips and a Carlton beer, which I enjoyed after the Kozzie summit, would be my reward, after a dip in the pool sounded refreshing. The outdoor pool was situated about 20 floors up. How do you think my vertigo did? High mountains, high bridges, and now high pools. I even managed a little nap poolside, but my red skin told me I overstayed my visit. How many Hoosiers get sunburned in January?

Monday, January 17, 2011

When departing from Sydney, I hoped to beat the morning rush hour traffic. A noble plan, but I was slow in its execution. I was ready, but waited for sunrise, thinking I could see better then. Unfortunately, that delay put me in the thick of traffic—and I do mean *thick*. These Aussie drivers were in a hurry. Traffic in my direction was five lanes wide. I tried not to creep, but I needed time to read the directional signs and react. I silenced my GPS to get out of Sydney and had the hotel print up a Mapquest info sheet. Having something on paper seemed reassuring.

With every glance at my paper map, I was honked at as I drove from downtown Sydney to its outskirts toward Melbourne. One irate driver was a motorcyclist who roared past me, leaned his bike into my lane directly in front of me, and popped his hand up to flip me the bird. All I could do was laugh and say, "If I were in your position, I'd probably flip me the bird too." The motorcyclist gave me a valuable lesson about being a more humble driver back home. I could drive more kindly. I didn't need to be a jerk. Not that I was a road rager, but I pledged to do better and be more courteous.

Somehow I made it out of Sydney's traffic—and then received another gift. Unknowingly, I had completely missed the signs for Melbourne, but I decided on a whim to take the next exit off the four lane road. I didn't need a restroom break or petrol. Honestly, it was one of those voice things, just like the voice that got me started on my Seven Summits quest. Something said: "Exit here—now!" And I did.

At the first intersection after that exit, I saw signs for Melbourne and made the appropriate turn. There are no coincidences in my book. I got off where I was supposed to get off, but only because I had "voice" help. I would have probably figured it out sooner or later without going on an Aussie walkabout. Nonetheless, I said a prayer of gratitude. "Voices—thank you! This is better than the GPS."

Soon I was driving on another four lane road, travelling across a high, flat tableland. The troublesome perception problems with vision in my left eye and steering wheel on right side of car continued. But the flat level stretches helped me improve. I continued as a work in progress right-side driver, with depth perception issues, plus humility.

When I began feeling sleepy I pulled the car off the highway into a kind of rest stop for a few minutes, planning to snooze. Seldom do I feel uncomfortable, as in wary, on my expeditions. But at that time I noticed something—something I didn't hear.

My radar went up. This particular pullout and its restroom were screened by a berm from the road so my vehicle and I weren't visible to motorists passing-by. Maybe I heard alarm bells, maybe it was because I was out of drinking water, maybe it was because it was too warm to nap. Whatever "it" was, I decided that leaving this spot now was a good idea. My "voice" worked overtime to rally me from sleepiness. I'll probably never know exactly what threat existed in that spot, but I'm glad I left.

I was hoping to find a quaint little village to stop in for a day or two. I saw a sign for something with "Snow" in the name, and while that sounded good, the signs pointed the wrong way and the town or city was long miles away from the turnoff. So, I pressed on, telling myself, "I haven't really prayed to land in a serene spot. And my blood sugar is telling me I need to eat something. So it's time to pray."

"Dear God, please hear my prayer to find a quiet little village I would like, and maybe that the village will like me, too. And if it isn't too much trouble, dear God may I find it soon." I prayed earnestly. A few miles went by. The next sign I saw was for Wangaratta, so I pointed my car down its highway.

Unknowingly, I had entered the high country of Victoria Province and what were called the Victorian Alps, or Australian Alps. This area included the Snowy Mountains, home to the Seven Summits' Kozzie. But my mountain of last week was many miles away from here. I hoped to find Wangaratta, and that it would not disappoint.

Sure enough, I arrived at Wangaratta and stopped at the Community Information Station. One of the hotels they recommended for my budget was the Ryley Motor Inn, which turned out to be across the street from a good-sized Catholic parish campus called St. Patrick's. The parish included a large church building, a chapel, a school, and even a combined retirement community-nursing home.

And Wangaratta had many restaurants, so I soon found food that helped me feel better. Wangaratta also featured walking paths a few blocks away from the motel, and the motel had an inviting pool surrounded by palm trees. Nearby were two rivers, the Owens and the King. Some hiking trails went out their way. Another trail went out of town in a different direction, an old railway bed reclaimed for runners, walkers, and bicyclists. The weather in January made it feel like temperate Florida. Downtown shops and restaurants were a ten minute walk away from the Ryley.

Best of all, the Ryley operators were friendly and hospitable. In answer to my prayer, I found a lovely place with agreeable people. My immediate plans: Take a dip in the pool after having a bite to eat, watch Australian Open Tennis matches on television, and consider a plan to make the 140 mile trip to Melbourne to attend the Aussie Tennis Open before leaving the country on Saturday. As this was Monday, I thought of the Rolling Stones song "Time Is On My Side."

My new friends, the proprietors at the Ryley, were so helpful. They landed me a place to stay in Melbourne which was the key to being at the Open. Again, thanked God for leading me to a tranquil spot on a huge continent, with townfolks as hospitable as Hoosiers.

After the busyness and hustle of mega-urban Sydney with all its people and traffic; after the all the aridness and flooding in this part of Australia, unhurried Wangaratta was a gift wrapped in peace and joy. "Centering down" is a Quaker term that involves holy silence as the source of the soul. After three long drives on the wrong side of the road, a kind of pilgrimage to the highest place in Australia, and climb to the top of the world's biggest bridge in one of the continent's largest cities, I definitely felt the need to center down in Wangaratta. Now I had time to enjoy what I call the sacrament of simplification.

Tuesday, January 18, 2011

After a good night's sleep, I found my Ryley room had a Gideon's Bible (as did the Vibe Hotel in Sydney). I used it instead of my mini Bible version, which contained only Psalms and the New Testament. I enjoyed being able to move about in a full-size book with both the Old and New Testaments. Next I picked up the Cherokee spiritual meditations of Joyce Sequichie Hifler, another wake-up practice I am vigilant about. Then, I updated my journal and reviewed the blog to help relieve my lonely feelings. Lori had posted there—smile.

Later, I strolled into downtown Wangaratta, located a restaurant, and have a huge breakfast with lots of java. I read a Melbourne newspaper, happy to be in a country where the papers were in English. Of course, upon arriving Down Under, I had to train my ears and brain to sort out the accent. The language in Aussie the paper did vary a bit from what I might read in *The Indianapolis Star* or *The Columbus Republic*. On my other expeditions I saw newspapers in Russian, Nepalese, and Swahili. Kathmandu did have one English newspaper.

I trained in journalism, so I appreciate reading a printed newspaper every morning. Digital papers don't quite get it for me, the dinosaur. Breakfast just seems better with a newspaper in front of me. It is my gateway to the world, especially since I haven't had a television since moving into my new home in May, 1998. Deleting television was one of the best decisions of my life. (Disclosure: Lori moved a TV set in with her in 2014.)

The Aussie Open just got started over the week end and I enjoy catching up on tournament play in the paper. I am amused that cricket matches and "football" (soccer) and rugby received equal news space with a world-wide Grand Slam tennis event. The reporting and writing style Down Under was different than what I learned at Ernie Pyle Hall and the School of Journalism at Indiana University, but it made for entertaining reading.

I cruised the downtown area, looking in shops windows, hearing people tell me "G'day" and "G'day mate" while smiling. In spite of all the people walking and traffic on the streets, no one showed any sign of being rushed. Wangaratta felt refreshing to me.

While walking back toward the Ryley, I crossed the street to visit the stately St. Patrick's Church. The door was unlocked—yes! The parish had a morning Mass, already ended. I knelt in a pew to say prayers and, as I learned from my Aunt Angie, I lighted candles for loved ones, both living and deceased. The strike of the match was the only sound in the chapel. While leaving the church, I spoke with a kindly parish worker about meeting the priest. "He'll be here for Mass tomorrow morning at eight o'clock," she told me. "Come 'round then, to the chapel next door."

Back at the hotel, I spoke with the proprietors Gill and Gloria about the Aussie Open. I told them, "I have no accommodations in Melbourne, I don't know my way around the city, and I'm only mediocre at getting about in the right-handed car. I want to see at least one day of play, maybe more. The cost of the hotel and the Open are considerations for my weary budget."

Gloria listened patiently and well, making a note or two. "Leave this with us. We know some hotel people in Melbourne. Check back."

She accomplished meeting my needs in no time. When I stopped after lunch she gave me the update. "I arranged a room at a nice motel on the outskirts of Melbourne. The tram, you call it a train, runs right in front of the hotel. You will board the train, do one changeover, and in 20 minutes you'll be standing on the grounds of the Australian Open."

"Oh, my gosh Gloria! Really?"

"I just need your credit card to hold the room," she said with a smile.

Done deal. "Thank you Gloria." And to myself I added, "And thanks, God, for such wonderful people."

Once again I was struck how lodgings and kindness unfolded as though someone were watching out for me. You think?

Many of my hospital colleagues have heard me ask: "What does calmness beget?"

A rare one knows the answer. When I say, "Calmness begets calmness," I saw their faces light up. I believe calmness is a way of being awake in the world. I believe most everyone in Wangaratta would know the answer to my "calmness" question. They seemed to inherently understand the Rule of St. Benedict about hospitality: "We are to treat others as though it is Christ himself."

I decided to spend the next few days centering down in Wangaratta, where I felt relaxed, and emotionally at ease. And now my body and mind and spirit were ready for what I love to do— exercise. Time for a walkabout, as the Australian Aborigines call it. For them the walkabout has deep and rich ancestral and spiritual roots. Such a journey can involve days, weeks, and even months. For them, the walkabout is a spiritual pilgrimage. I told myself that walking Down Under gave me at least a remote connection with the aboriginals who had walked hereabouts.

And today I found a grassy spot that actually was hallowed aboriginal ground. A historical marker advised me the area I trekked past was a primitive aboriginal gathering ground. The area I stood beside had been a kind of sanctuary land for them as this rural white pioneer village began to develop.

For me, 20 minutes of walking equals one mile. I stayed in motion with my backpack on for almost seven miles, or 140 minutes. My walkabout followed a creek and I went outbound for half of it, then turned and retraced my steps. Under bridges where the trail came close to the creek, I stayed wary of the water. After all, Australia does have crocs—and those deadly spiders. In certain spots I had to detour around high water caused by the rains and flooding.

The trek took me past the public tennis courts—grass courts. Public grass tennis courts are unimaginable back home. The expense and the maintenance of upkeep would badly undermine the budget of a public park and recreation department. I love playing tennis, but there I was in trek boots and a backpack, without a racquet or tennis shoes. I've always dreamed of playing tennis on a grass surface. Synthetic grass on a private court in South Carolina is as close as I've gotten.

I let myself inside one of the gates for the four courts. Now I was walking on a grass court. Three young adults on one court were having much fun playing two verses one—a game I taught my friends at Donner Park in Columbus on what I thought of as my home court. I called it "Italian Doubles." The singles player competes against two opponents, using doubles rules, while they play singles rules against him. It helps with skill development and the game is a vigorous competitive workout.

As for me, simply feeling the tennis court grass under my trek boots was the best of both worlds—trekking and tennis. The day's exercise ended back at the Ryley Motel. My Blackberry registered a call from Lori, and all was well.

For the third day in a row I swam and sunned myself, still finding this remarkable in January. Snow and ice collected at home, Lori said. Here, the pool deck was too hot under my butt, so I alternated between a chair, and siting directly on the deck surface after splashing water to cool the hot surface. I considered putting my chair in the pool but it seemed a little over the top, and I didn't want to tear the pool liner. I did laundry using the pool water and hung out my hand-dipped trek duds to dry on the pool chairs.

My journal records that I felt: "Content, Grateful, Expectant, Homesick, and Hungry."

Later, I bought carry-out fish and chips and ate while watching Australian Open tennis on television. Thanks to Gloria, on Thursday I would drive 2.5 hours to my new digs in Melbourne at the St. Georges Motor Inn, and then be just a 20 minute tram ride from the real deal of Grand Slam tennis action.

Wednesday, January 19, 2011

This day started the same as Tuesday when I awakened at 4:15 a.m. After reading scripture, I updated the 2Trek4Kids blog and then walked to St. Patrick's Church where I attended Mass, received Holy Communion, and met the priest. He commended the mountain climbing and youth obesity fund raising initiative with a hearty "Good on ya!"

I trekked another six miles, or two hours, much of it along the old railway bed turned into a rails-to-trails path connecting Wangaratta to nearby towns. I talked with Lori again—nice to do that for two days in a row. Hearing her cheerful voice helped with my homesickness. I dipped in the pool again and visited with a guy who bicycled the trail in. Later, I packed my gear for an early departure the next morning, and the walked downtown to buy fish and chips and a cold Carlton beer before returning to the hotel to watch tennis. And to bed.

Thursday, January 20, 2016

At 5 a.m. the tele rang with a wake-up call from Gloria. I had rolled over a few seconds before to check my clock. I thanked Gloria and told her, "The Ryley and Wangaratta will always have a place in my heart."

Today my third Down Under dream would unfold—Grand Slam Tennis. But first I needed to get my butt to the St. George for my pre-arranged early room check in. Tennis matches begin at 11 a.m. Would I reach the Rod Laver Arena before the first tennis ball was struck in match play?

My GPS Commander and I travelled in harmony most of the way to Melbourne. Somehow I made two wrong turns, but with GPS "recalculating" support, I found my way to the the St. Georges Motor Inn by 9:30 a.m. I parked the car, and walked in the front door to see a pleasant face and heard a cordial voice say, "You must be Walter." Cool to be expected, what?

When I returned in a few minutes, Joseph handed me a paper. "Here's a tram map with all the routes and the times. The tram will be out front in just a few minutes. I've marked your route. You only have one change-over, here," he showed me on the map. He told me how to pay for tokens for the tram. "Do you have any questions?"

It all seemed so simple, but I felt a little overwhelmed. Not seeing the tram track, I said, "Now where's the pick-up?"

Joseph smiled, led me outside, and walked me to the platform. "Have fun. See you later in the day!"

Minutes later the tram came, and off I went. I counted Joseph's organization and hospitality as another in the long list of kindnesses I received on this trip.

I saw the sights as we rolled into downtown Melbourne—another mega-city. In the heart of downtown Melbourne I spotted a St. Vincent Hospital. I knew it was there, but still I rubbed my eyes. I wished I had time to drop by and say "hello" from the American branch of the international St. Vincent healthcare family.

In about 20 minutes I was on the grounds of the Australian Open and had purchased my admission ticket. Then I was standing in front of The Rod Laver Arena complete with big sign. And I arrived well before match play began.

You may be wondering, "Who is Rod Laver, for whom the arena is named?" Arguably, he is the finest player ever to play the game of tennis. From Australia, he is a legend among legends. And I met him a couple of times.

I met Rod Laver in Indianapolis through St. Vincent Hospital's connection to the RCA Hard Courts Tennis Championship. This event brought many of the best male players in the world to Indy for a competition two weeks before the United States Tennis Open Championships in New York City, another of the four Grand Slams. What a thrill to meet Rod Laver, affectionately called "Rocket."

Rod was at the center of a teaching and exhibition morning event on the clay courts at the Indy Tennis Center in downtown where the RCA event was held. He amicably chatted with visitors between sessions, shaking hands and signing autographs with great patience. I walked over and chatted him up a bit. He was low-key, un-assuming, and friendly. Also sweaty from having taught and played tennis. But mostly, I found him to be genuinely friendly. He was my tennis hero, and I told him I followed his career and was a big fan. He was humble.

He wore an RCA Hard Courts hat with a sweat stain ringing the brim. Later in the week I snagged a pair of his Reebox tennis shoes through a silent auction. Rod's autographed shoes, which by the way fit me perfectly, are among my prize tennis possessions.

The Rocket and I met a second time at the hard courts a couple years later. Before becoming a chaplain with St. Vincent, I recruited physicians for them. One of my specialized assignments was finding a pediatric ophthalmologist, and I was blessed to find a real winner in a woman whose training, competency, and personality resonated with our practice physicians. She came to Indianapolis and visited the hospital, the practice, and the family's home for dinner. Her visit to Indy concluded on a Saturday morning but her plane didn't depart until the afternoon.

The RCA Hard Courts were occurring and I knew the physician enjoyed tennis, so I suggested I'd collect her early, we could attend a few matches, and then I'd drop her at the airport. With St. Vincent as an event sponsor, I procured great seats a few rows above the court surface, next to the players' entrance to the court. A good match was going on and the weather was ideal. Our seats next to the players' entrance were at a perfect level to see the players come and go, as well as the on-going match. A small group of people sauntered up to watch the match, and who did I spy but Rod Laver. I caught his eye and nodded a big hello. He walked over to us and I told him I was one of hundreds of fans he'd met here in Indy. I was pleased to introduce our physician recruit, who shook hands with the legend and basked in the warmth of his charming, ebullient personality. I asked him to autograph a program for her, which he did with a smile.

And now here I was in Melbourne, Australia, standing in front of Rod Laver Arena. Rod was the first man to win all four grand slam tournaments (Aussie, Wimbledon in England, French and U.S.) in one calendar year and wasn't he the only man to do so twice. A tremendous competitor in both singles and doubles, he exhibited joy whenever he played.

My dollars were draining. A night at the St. George was $125, and the Aussie Open was $135, with ticket upgrades available—for more bucks of course. I finally shrugged and told myself, "To heck with It! Enjoy yourself, because you'll not be back this way again."

I had time to visit several practice courts before the morning's warm-up concluded and competitive play began. Though I didn't recognize many players' names in opening round play, I do recognize tennis talent. And I saw a lot of talent—such power, athleticism, and reactions. Just strolling these grounds sent a thrill up my spine. I walked among bronze busts of Australia's best men and women players in a heritage courtyard. That was breathtaking.

I found a seat in Margaret Court Arena and, as I took my place, heard many languages spoken. Each player had a partisan chorus from his or her own country. Not only vocal cheers, but hand clapping and people using their hands to thump on the chairs around them. An orderly ruckus prevailed, with the crowd self-suspending noise during actual points, per tennis etiquette. The first match included an Israeli woman whose crew waved a huge national flag on a pole with a blue Star of David on a white background between points. Her fans wore Israeli headbands. I enjoyed the match for several games, even though I didn't know the players.

The day was hot, though it could have been worse. At times the court temperatures would reach 130 degrees Fahrenheit. An upgraded ticket would let me enter the indoor, climate-controlled Laver Stadium, but I passed on it. I got myself a cold beer and strolled around the grounds, visiting other venues and matches; taking in all courts my ticket entitles me to. On one of about 30 side courts I watched an exciting women's doubles match from the second row. The passionate family of one of the players sat on the front row right in front of me. After watching tennis for several hours, I believed I had one great day at my first and only Grand Slam Event. And, I was wilted too.

Heading back to the St. Georges, a surprise awaited me. First I boarded the wrong tram. Where was my GPS Commander when

I needed her? The "wrong" tram took me past St Paul's Cathedral in downtown Melbourne! "Oh, happy fault!" as is written about Adam and Eve's transgression in the Garden of Eden. My tram miscue paid a huge dividend as I got off and walked into a historic and beautiful Anglican Cathedral. The stained glass front doors were huge, imposing yet welcoming. Stained glass windows inside the church were among the tallest I'd ever seen. I remember it as the oldest church in Melbourne, located almost in the heart of the city. A worship guide flier said the day's service would remember Australian flood victims.

In 1835, the church marked the first Christian service in Melbourne. Like America's National Cathedral (also Anglican-sponsored) in Washington, D.C., it was built in stages over several decades. As an example, when I checked dates, the cathedral was consecrated 120 years and one day before my visit. By contrast, the spires were not begun until 1926. The cathedral maintains the English tradition of a choral—an evening prayer rendered in music. It is the only church in Australia observing this custom, which reminded me of the daily evening practice at my seminary St. Meinrad, where the prayer service including music and readings is called vespers.

I walked about the church in awe. Going from the sunlight and heat to dark and some cool made me feel light-headed. I drank water, which helped.

Time to head back to Joseph and his St. Georges Motor Inn for my last comfortable night in Australia. Upon arrival, I thanked Joseph for helping set up a wonderful day. He gave me directions to a fish and chips place where I ordered (what else?) fish and chips, and a salad. The fish and chips came wrapped in newspaper, as is the local custom. I still hadn't overdosed on tennis, so back in my room I turned on the telly and watched evening matches.

Friday, January 21, 2011

Scripture and fervent prayers followed the wake up alarm. I wanted to be God-centered before I popped out of bed. My prayers were succinct:

"Thank you God for this adventure. I ask you to bless Lori, my sons, their families, Lori's daughters and family including Gloria her mom, and all our loved ones. Please bless our youth obesity patients and families, their clinicians, and our donors.

"Thank you, creator God, for my body, mind and spirit; Jesus for your atoning sacrifice to make my earthen vessel body worthy; and, in Cherokee, Galun Lati Great Holy Spirit I thank you for your timeless promises to me and my loved ones. Help me and each of us greet the new sun with confidence that this will be the best day of my and our lives." (This last sentence was courtesy of Og Mandino).

A shower felt good, and I realized the hair gel I brought to Australia was an Aussie Aussome Volume product, purchased in Columbus, Indiana.

The drive to the Melbourne International Airport was uneventful, even with the heavy traffic. Joseph prepped me with excellent directions. And God's angels were, as I asked, a hedge about me, today, as they were throughout the trip. All went smoothly except for some sweaty palms.

Lori called about a milli-second before I reached for the tele to call her! We had a lovely catch-up visit. She had new youth obesity patients that day at Peyton Manning Children's Hospital and was driving home in a snowfall.

Her final words to me: "Come home! Your work in Australia is done."

And I agreed. At the airport, I met a waiter at the restaurant from the States. Closer conversation revealed he was from Indiana.

Not only that, he was an Avon High School graduate. What were the chances? Brad was seeing the world, but hadn't been able to save much money in Melbourne because expenses were so high. He planned to come back to Indiana within a month or two. In addition to a tip I slip him a little extra cash—call it Hoosier hospitality exported to Australia.

Like Brad, my expenses ran high. I exchanged all my Australian dollars except for one souvenir Australian $5 bill with the Queen's pleasant countenance gracing it. With reserves dwindled, rather than getting a room, I choose to be a vagabond my last night in Australia. I slept on an airport bench after checking my bags for safekeeping. Most all the bench space around me was similarly used. I laughed at one neighbor who carried a half-deflated basketball. He noted in Australian tones, it was easier to travel with the ball that way. I told him "Where I come from, those are king." He didn't seem interested. Selfishly, I was kind of glad. I needed sleep, not hoops talk.

Saturday, January 22, 2011

Departure day dawned and I used my final Aussie dollars for a great cup of coffee at McDonald's. The Melbourne flight to Los Angeles went without a hitch, as did the LAX leg to Dallas-Fort Worth. Then came the "Oops." One plane hop away from home at Dallas-Fort Worth, I boarded my last flight, buckled in, and then learned the brakes on the plane were bad.

"Why in the world did they load us?" I groused. That kind of defect would have shown in pre-flight checks surely. Finally, the airline secures another plane. We boarded, and finally headed for Indy. My seatmate was an Indianapolis physician, recently widowed, whose wife was at the St. Vincent Hospice. I ministered to him and he ministers to me also, as I felt a little nauseous. He was fascinated by my Seven Summits quest.

This final flight went quickly and soon I saw the light of Indy below. Next, I saw the welcoming glow in Lori's eyes. Somehow, she received TSA permission to meet me right at my gate as I deplaned. It felt so good to be with her—and great to be home. I could hardly wait to see my sons and families. But first I saw— snow! At midnight we parked in the white stuff in front of the Columbus Kroger Store so I could get comfort food. Fried chicken and mashed potatoes at midnight; that's how I wrapped up 12 days in Australia.

Ah, back home again in Indiana!

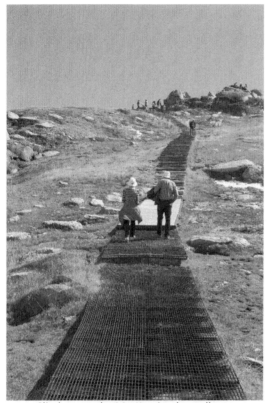

Climbers on the Mt. Kosciuszko walkway

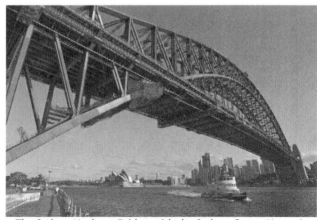

The Sydney Harbour Bridge with the Sydney Opera House in background

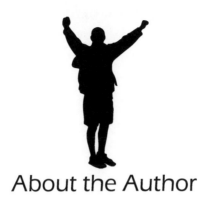

About the Author

Since turning age 59 in 2007, Walter Glover has climbed on five of the Seven Summits, the highest mountains on each of the seven continents, Mount Rainier twice, and trekked along most of the 490 mile pilgrimage across Spain The Way of St. James, El Camino. A pastoral care hospital chaplain, Walter's expeditions raised $130,000 for St. Vincent Hospitals to help fight childhood obesity in southern Indiana.

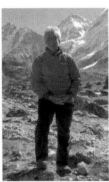

Walter with Mt. Everest over his left shoulder.

The quest was for all the Seven Summits, but that dream was re-imagined after a fall on Mount Rainier showed Walter suffered from three aneurysms in three separate body systems, a medical rarity. One of the aneurysms required open heart surgery. Heart disease had claimed his father and brother early in life.

Glover retired from St. Vincent Hospitals in southern Indiana at age 65. The father of two and grandfather of two, he makes his home in Columbus, Indiana.

Glover has worked as a professional award winning journalist, and also holds a Master's Degree in Theologic Studies from St.

Meinrad Seminary. He is a certified grief counselor. When not on expedition, his retirement activities include providing bereavement support to three groups, including bereft parents.

These compelling stories from the mountains are told from the perspective of wellness advocate, senior citizen, world traveler, heart surgery survivor, theologian, grief counselor, adventurer and mountaineer, and family man.

Walter's treks and climbs support The Foundation for Youth
If you'd like to donate . . .

Checks should be made payable (and mailed) to:

The Foundation for Youth
405 Hope Avenue,
Columbus IN 47201

Please include your name, complete address, phone number, and email address (to receive blog updates and photos from Walter's treks).

Check Memo Line: Scholarships / 2Trek4Kids

For credit card donations, go to www.foundationforyouth.com and click "Donations" to make credit card gift to Scholarships / 2trek4kids.

All contributions are tax deductible to the maximum extent allowed by law.

"There are no finish lines for kids," Glover says about his collaboration with Foundation for Youth. "Wellness initiatives don't need to come to an end even if you're age 69. There's no finish line when it comes to helping kids become physically, emotionally, mentally and spiritually fit so as to become well-integrated adults."

The Foundation for Youth

In Columbus, Indiana, **The Foundation for Youth** exists to serve youth and the community by supporting many valuable programs and services. Your donation will help provide—

- A safe environment for children to work, play, and grow
- Life-enhancing programs designed to educate and provide skills to succeed in life,
- Relationships with caring, trained adults who are responsive to a child's daily realities.

Groups supported by the program include the Boys and Girls Club, Columbus Youth Camp, Big Brothers-Big Sisters, Communities That Care, Police Athletic Activities League, and many more.

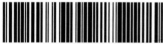

Printed in Great Britain
by Amazon